Gluten-Free & Dairy-Free Cookbook

Easy and Satisfying Recipes with No Gluten and No Dairy.

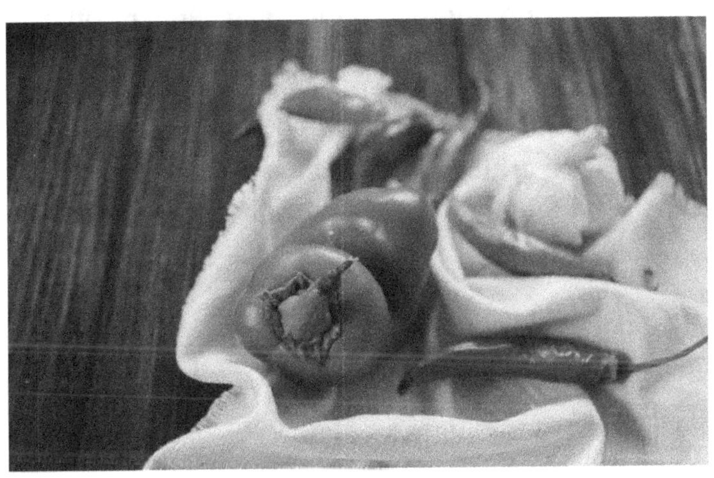

Thelma Howard

TABLE OF CONTENTS

INTRODUCTION

In the quaint town of Culinary Haven, where aromas danced through the air, lived Chef Thelma. Known for her culinary wizardry, she faced a peculiar challenge – creating dishes that catered to the growing demand for gluten-free and dairy-free alternatives. Determined to weave a tapestry of flavors accessible to all, she embarked on a journey that would redefine the town's gastronomic landscape.

Chef Thelma's Gluten-Free & Dairy-Free Cookbook is a testament to her creative prowess, offering a symphony of recipes that transcended dietary restrictions. Each page unfolds a culinary adventure, guiding readers through a world where dietary limitations become a canvas for delectable masterpieces.

From the crisp pages emanates the aroma of freshly baked bread without gluten's grip and creamy delights absent of dairy's influence. Chef Thelma's cookbook isn't just a collection of recipes; it's a celebration of inclusivity, proving that flavor knows no bounds.

As the townsfolk eagerly flipped through the cookbook, Culinary Haven embraced a new era of gastronomy. Chef Thelma's creations not only satisfied the palates of those with dietary sensitivities but also won the hearts of everyone who dared to embark on this culinary expedition.

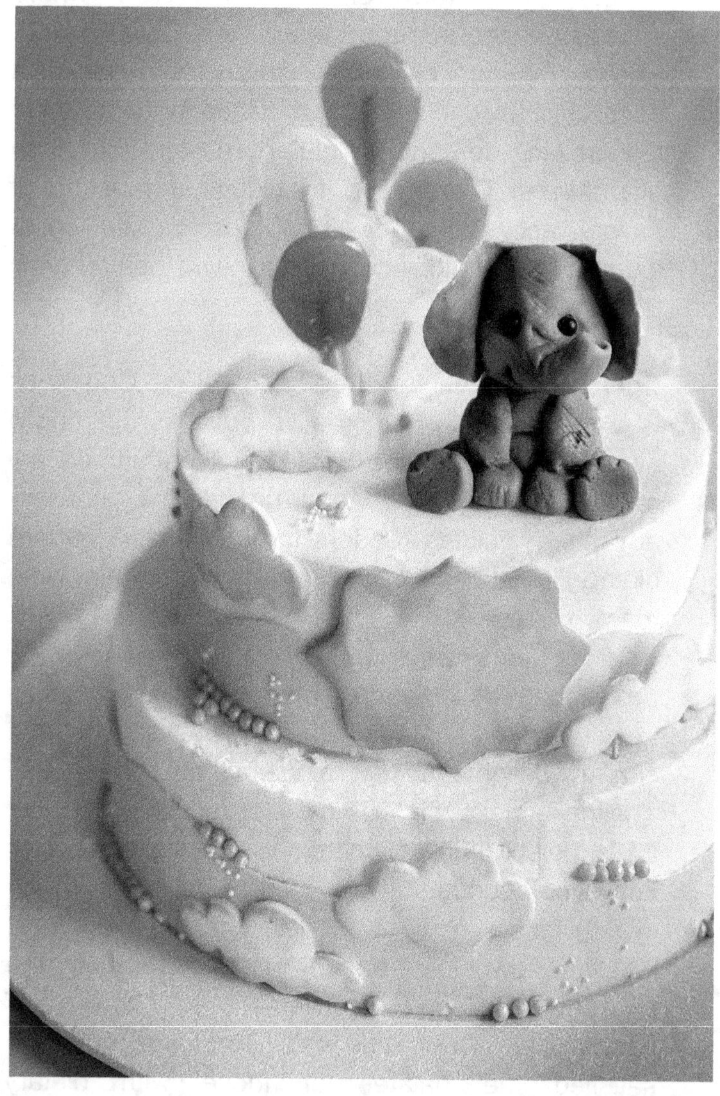

CHAPTER ONE

Gluten-Free and Diary-Free Lifestyle

Living a gluten-free lifestyle means avoiding foods that contain gluten, a protein found in wheat, barley, and rye. For those with celiac disease or gluten sensitivity, consuming gluten can lead to digestive issues and other health complications. Gluten-free living involves choosing alternative grains like rice, quinoa, and corn, and opting for gluten-free versions of products.

On the other hand, a dairy-free lifestyle involves avoiding dairy products due to lactose intolerance or dairy allergies. Dairy-free living means steering clear of milk, cheese, yogurt, and other products derived from cow's milk. Almond, soy, coconut, and oat milk are popular dairy alternatives.

Benefits of Gluten-Free and Diary-Free Living

The benefits of gluten-free and dairy-free living extend beyond catering to specific health conditions. Many individuals report increased energy levels, improved digestion, and better skin health when adopting these dietary changes. Gluten-free diets can be especially crucial for those with celiac disease, preventing long-term damage to the small intestine.

Dairy-free living can alleviate symptoms like bloating, gas, and digestive discomfort for those who are lactose intolerant. Additionally, some people choose these diets as a lifestyle choice, believing it contributes to overall well-being.
Both gluten-free and dairy-free living often require careful label reading and mindful food choices. While these diets offer health benefits for some, it's essential to ensure a well-balanced nutritional intake, seeking guidance from healthcare professionals or nutritionists when making significant dietary changes.

Living a gluten-free and dairy-free lifestyle involves careful attention to ingredients and a proactive approach to prevent cross-contamination and accidental exposure. Here's a comprehensive overview:

Gluten-Free Ingredients:
1. Gluten-Free Grains:
   - Opt for alternatives like rice, quinoa, corn, and gluten-free oats.
   - Use flours made from almonds, coconut, or chickpeas for baking.

2. Proteins:
   - Choose fresh meats, fish, and poultry in their natural state.

- Be cautious with processed meats and deli items, as they might contain gluten-containing additives.

3. Fruits and Vegetables:
    - Fresh fruits and vegetables are naturally gluten-free.
    - Be cautious with canned or frozen varieties, checking for added ingredients.

4. Dairy Alternatives:
    - Opt for non-dairy milk like almond, soy, coconut, or oat milk.
    - Look for dairy-free alternatives for cheese and yogurt.

Dairy-Free Ingredients:
1. Milk Alternatives:
    - Choose plant-based milks like almond, soy, rice, or oat milk.
    - Coconut and cashew milk are also popular dairy-free options.

2. Non-Dairy Yogurt and Cheese:
    - Explore alternatives made from soy, almond, or coconut for yogurt.
    - Dairy-free cheese options include those made from nuts, soy, or tapioca.

3. Butter Substitutes:
    - Use plant-based spreads or oils like olive oil, coconut oil, or avocado oil.

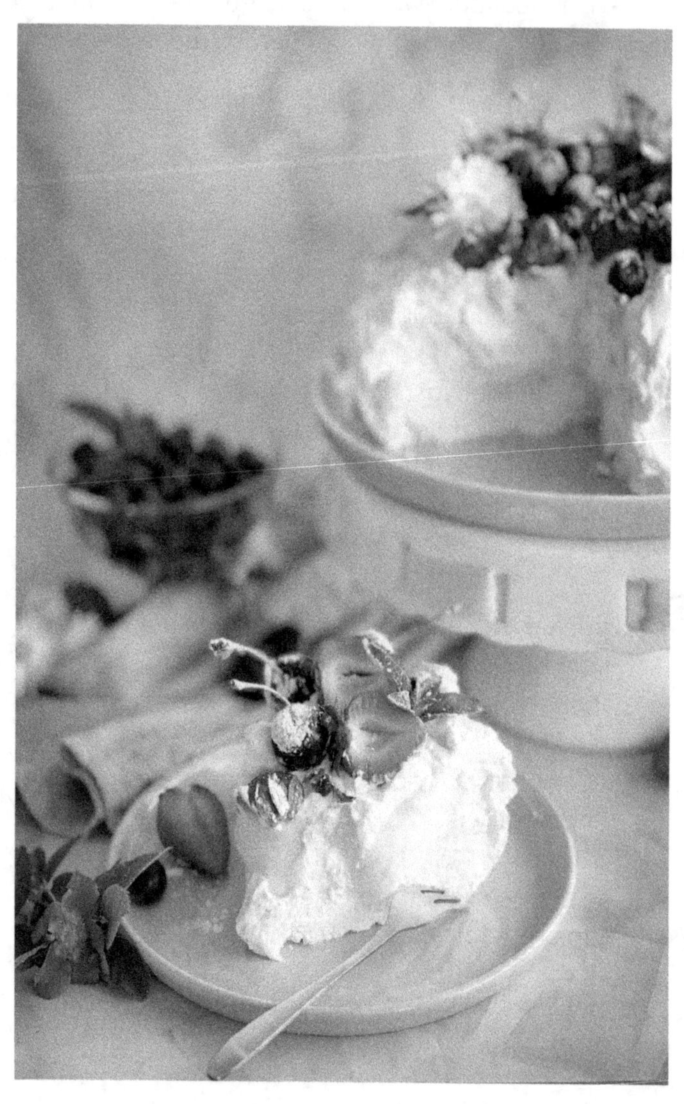

CHAPTER TWO

Breakfast

Creating delicious and nutritious gluten-free and dairy-free breakfasts requires a thoughtful selection of ingredients and a bit of creativity. Here's a comprehensive guide to some enticing breakfast recipes:

1. Gluten-Free Oatmeal:

Making gluten-free oatmeal is a simple and delicious process.Use certified gluten-free oats. Top with fresh fruits, nuts, seeds, and a drizzle of honey or maple syrup. Here's a basic recipe for preparing gluten-free oatmeal:

Ingredients:
- 1 cup certified gluten-free rolled oats
- 2 cups dairy-free milk (almond, coconut, soy, etc.)
- Sweeteners like agave, maple syrup, or honey are optional.

- Toppings: Fresh fruits, nuts, seeds, or dried fruits

Instructions:
1. Choose Certified Gluten-Free Oats:
    - Ensure that the oats are labeled as "certified gluten-free" to avoid any cross-contamination during processing.

2. Combine Oats and Dairy-Free Milk:
   - In a saucepan, combine 1 cup of certified gluten-free rolled oats with 2 cups of your preferred dairy-free milk.

3. Cook on the Stovetop:
   - Over medium heat, bring the mixture to a mild boil, stirring from time to time.

4. Simmer:
   -Once the oats are soft, reduce the heat to low and simmer for five to seven minutes. Stir occasionally to prevent sticking.

5. Sweeten to Taste:
   - Add sweeteners like honey, maple syrup, or agave to taste. Adapt according to your desired level of sweetness.

6. Top with Your Favorites:
   - Take the oats off the stove as soon as it reaches the consistency you prefer.

   - Serve in bowls and top with your favorite gluten-free and dairy-free toppings, such as fresh fruits, nuts, seeds, or dried fruits.

Additional Tips:
Gluten-Free Toppings:
   - Ensure that the toppings you choose are gluten-free. Fresh fruits, sliced bananas, berries, or chopped nuts are excellent choices.

- Experiment with Flavors:
  - Enhance the flavor by adding a dash of cinnamon, vanilla extract, or a sprinkle of coconut flakes.

- Make It Creamier:
  - If you prefer creamier oatmeal, use more dairy-free milk or even add a scoop of dairy-free yogurt.

- **Microwave Option**:
  - If you're short on time, you can also make gluten-free oatmeal in the microwave. Combine oats and dairy-free milk in a microwave-safe bowl and heat in 30-second increments, stirring in between until it reaches your desired consistency.

Enjoy your gluten-free oatmeal as a warm and comforting breakfast, customized with your favorite flavors and toppings!

2. Quinoa Breakfast Bowl:

Creating a quinoa breakfast bowl is a nutritious and versatile option. Here is a basic recipe to help you along:

Ingredients:
- 1 cup quinoa (rinsed)
- 2 cups water or dairy-free milk (almond, coconut, soy, etc.)

- 1-2 tablespoons sweetener (honey, maple syrup, or agave), optional
- Toppings: Fresh fruits, nuts, seeds, coconut flakes, or dairy-free yogurt

Instructions:
1. Rinse Quinoa:
  - Use cold water to rinse one cup of quinoa to get rid of any bitterness.
2. Cook Quinoa:
  - In a saucepan, combine the rinsed quinoa with 2 cups of water or dairy-free milk.
3. Bring to a Boil:
  - Using a medium-high heat setting, bring the mixture to a boil.
4. Simmer:
  - Reduce the heat to low, cover the saucepan, and let it simmer for about 15-20 minutes or until the quinoa is cooked and the liquid is absorbed.
5. Fluff Quinoa:
  Use a fork to fluff the cooked quinoa..
6. Sweeten to Taste:
  - Add sweeteners like honey, maple syrup, or agave if desired. Adjust according to your sweetness preference.
7. Assemble Breakfast Bowl:
  - Spoon the cooked quinoa into bowls.
8. Add Toppings:
  - Top the quinoa with your favorite gluten-free and dairy-free toppings. Options include fresh fruits (berries, sliced banana), nuts (almonds, walnuts),

seeds (chia seeds, flaxseeds), coconut flakes, or a dollop of dairy-free yogurt.

Additional Tips:
Experiment with Spices:
   - Enhance the flavor of your quinoa by adding spices like cinnamon, nutmeg, or vanilla extract.

Texture Variation:
   - Play with textures by adding crunchy toppings like granola or toasted coconut.

Prep Ahead:
   - Cook a batch of quinoa ahead of time and store it in the fridge. In the morning, simply reheat and add your toppings for a quick and convenient breakfast.

Protein Boost:
   - Incorporate a scoop of dairy-free protein powder or nut butter for an added protein boost.

This quinoa breakfast bowl provides a hearty and nutritious start to your day, and the customization options make it a versatile and enjoyable breakfast choice.
Cook quinoa and top with berries, sliced bananas, and a dollop of almond or coconut yogurt.

3. **Chia Seed Pudding**:
Making chia seed pudding is a simple and healthy way to start your day. Basic recipe:

Ingredients:
- 1/4 cup chia seeds
- 1 cup dairy-free milk (almond, coconut, soy, etc.)
- 1-2 tablespoons sweetener (honey, maple syrup, or agave), optional
- 1/2 teaspoon vanilla extract (optional)
- Toppings: Fresh fruits, nuts, or seeds

Instructions:
1. Mix Chia Seeds and Liquid:
   - In a bowl or jar, combine 1/4 cup of chia seeds with 1 cup of your preferred dairy-free milk.
2. Stir Well:
   - Stir the mixture well to ensure that the chia seeds are evenly distributed in the liquid.
3. Sweeten and Flavor:
   - Add sweeteners like honey, maple syrup, or agave to taste. You can also include vanilla extract for added flavor if desired.
4. Let it Sit:
   - Cover the bowl or jar and refrigerate for at least 2 hours or preferably overnight. The liquid will be absorbed by the chia seeds, giving the mixture a pudding-like consistency.
5. Stir Again:
   - After the initial setting time, give the mixture a good stir to break up any clumps and ensure a smooth texture.
6. Check Consistency:
   - If the pudding is too thick, you can add more dairy-free milk to reach your desired consistency.

7. Top with Toppings:
    - When ready to serve, add your favorite gluten-free and dairy-free toppings such as fresh fruits, nuts, or seeds.

Additional Tips:
Experiment with Flavors:
  - Customize your chia seed pudding by adding flavors like cocoa powder, cinnamon, or a hint of citrus zest.

Texture Variation:
  - Include crunchy toppings like chopped nuts or granola for added texture.

Prep Ahead:
  - Make a batch the night before for a quick and convenient breakfast option.

Play with Ratios:
  - Adjust the chia seed to liquid ratio based on your desired thickness.

Chia seed pudding is not only a delicious and satisfying breakfast but also a versatile dish that allows for creativity with flavors and toppings.

4. **Smoothie Bowl**:
Creating a delicious and nutritious smoothie bowl is quick and easy. Blend frozen fruits, non-dairy milk,

and a handful of spinach or kale. Top with gluten-free granola, coconut flakes, and chia seeds. Here's a simple recipe to guide

Ingredients:
- 1 frozen banana
-One cup of frozen raspberries, blueberries, and strawberries
- 1/2 cup dairy-free milk (almond, coconut, soy, etc.)
- Toppings: Fresh fruits, nuts, seeds, granola, or coconut flakes

Instructions:
1. Blend the Smoothie Base:
   - In a blender, combine the frozen banana, frozen berries, and dairy-free milk.
2. Blend Until Smooth:
   - Blend the ingredients until you achieve a smooth and thick consistency. You may need to pause and scrape down the sides as needed.
3. Adjust Consistency:
   - If the smoothie is too thick, you can add more dairy-free milk in small increments until you reach your desired thickness.
4. Pour into a Bowl:
   Transfer the blended drink to a bowl.
5. Add Toppings:
   - Top your smoothie bowl with a variety of gluten-free and dairy-free toppings. This can include fresh fruits (sliced banana, berries), nuts

(almonds, walnuts), seeds (chia seeds, flaxseeds), granola, or coconut flakes.

6. Arrange Toppings Creatively:

- Arrange the toppings in an aesthetically pleasing manner for a visually appealing breakfast.

Additional Tips:

Experiment with Flavors:

- Add ingredients like spinach or kale for a green smoothie bowl, or include a scoop of dairy-free protein powder for an extra boost.

Texture Variation:

- Include a mix of crunchy and chewy toppings for a satisfying texture.

Prep Ahead:

- Prepare smoothie packs by portioning out frozen fruits in advance for a quick and convenient breakfast.

Customize to Taste:

- Adjust the sweetness by adding natural sweeteners like honey, maple syrup, or agave if desired.

Smoothie bowls are not only a healthy and refreshing breakfast option but also offer endless possibilities for creativity and personalization. Enjoy your colorful and nutrient-packed creation!

5. **Avocado Toast on Gluten-Free Bread:**

Avocado toast on gluten-free bread is a simple yet delicious and nutritious breakfast or snack. Mash

avocado and spread it on gluten-free toast. Season with red pepper flakes, salt, and pepper.
Here's a step-by-step guide:

Ingredients:
- 1 ripe avocado
- 2 slices gluten-free bread
- Salt and pepper to taste
- Optional toppings: Red pepper flakes, cherry tomatoes, poached egg, or a drizzle of olive oil

Instructions:
1. Select Gluten-Free Bread:
   - Choose your favorite gluten-free bread. There are various options available, such as rice, quinoa, or almond flour-based bread.

2. Toast the Gluten-Free Bread:
   - Toast the slices of gluten-free bread in a toaster or on a grill until they reach your desired level of crispiness.

3. Prepare the Avocado:
   - Slice the ripe avocado in half while the bread is browning. After removing the pit, transfer the meat to a bowl..

4. Mash the Avocado:
   - Use a fork to mash the avocado until you achieve your preferred level of smoothness. Add salt and pepper to taste.

5. Spread Avocado on Toast:
   - Once the gluten-free bread is toasted, spread the mashed avocado evenly on each slice.

6. Season to Taste:
   -Sprinkle a touch extra salt and pepper over the avocado. You can also add red pepper flakes for a hint of spice.

7. Optional Toppings:
   - Get creative with toppings. Consider adding sliced cherry tomatoes, a poached egg, or a drizzle of olive oil for extra flavor and variety.

8. Serve and Enjoy:
   - Your avocado toast on gluten-free bread is ready to be enjoyed! For the most flavor and texture, serve it right away.

Additional Tips:

Fresh Ingredients:
  - Use ripe avocados for optimal creaminess and flavor.

Experiment with Flavors:
   - Try adding a squeeze of lime juice, balsamic glaze, or your favorite herbs for extra taste.

Protein Boost:
  - Include a protein element, like a poached egg, to make your avocado toast more filling.

Prep Ahead:

  - Prepare the mashed avocado ahead of time and store it in an airtight container in the fridge for a quick and convenient breakfast.

Avocado toast on gluten-free bread is a versatile dish that allows for personalization based on your preferences and dietary needs. Enjoy this nutritious and satisfying meal!

6. **Buckwheat Pancakes**:

  Making buckwheat pancakes is a delightful way to enjoy a gluten-free breakfast. Make pancakes using buckwheat flour. Top with dairy-free butter, pure maple syrup, and berries.
Here's a straightforward recipe that you can use:

Ingredients:
- 1 cup buckwheat flour
- 1 tablespoon sugar (or sweetener of choice)
- 1 teaspoon baking powder
- 1/2 teaspoon baking soda
- 1/4 teaspoon salt
- 1 cup dairy-free milk (almond, coconut, soy, etc.)
- 1 large egg (or flaxseed egg for an egg-free option)
- 2 tablespoons melted coconut oil or vegetable oil
- Optional: Vanilla extract, cinnamon, or nutmeg for added flavor

Instructions:
1. Combine Dry Ingredients:
   - In a mixing bowl, whisk together the buckwheat flour, sugar, baking powder, baking soda, and salt.

2. Prepare Wet Ingredients:
   - In a separate bowl, whisk together the dairy-free milk, egg (or flaxseed egg), melted coconut oil, and any optional flavorings like vanilla extract or spices.

3. Combine Wet and Dry Ingredients:
   Mixing until just mixed, pour the wet components into the dry ingredients. A few lumps are acceptable because overmixing can change the pancakes' texture.

4. Let the Batter Rest:
   Let the batter sit for ten minutes or so. This helps the buckwheat flour absorb the liquid and gives you fluffier pancakes.

5. Heat the Pan:
   Heat a griddle or nonstick skillet to medium. Use some cooking spray or oil.

6. Cook the Pancakes:
   - Pour 1/4 cup portions of batter onto the hot skillet. Cook until surface bubbles appear, then turn and continue cooking until golden brown on the other side.

7. Repeat:
   - Repeat the process until all the batter is used, adjusting the heat if needed to prevent burning.

8. Serve Warm:
   - Stack the pancakes on a plate and serve warm.

Additional Tips:
Toppings:
   - Top your buckwheat pancakes with fresh fruit, dairy-free yogurt, maple syrup, or a sprinkle of chopped nuts.

Texture Variation:
   - For added texture, consider incorporating ingredients like blueberries or chopped nuts into the batter.

Customize Flavors:
   - Experiment with flavors by adding ingredients like cinnamon, nutmeg, or a touch of citrus zest.

Make Ahead:
   - Cooked pancakes can be stored in the fridge or freezer and reheated for a quick breakfast on busy mornings.

Enjoy your delicious and gluten-free buckwheat pancakes!

7. **Coconut Flour Waffles**:
Creating coconut flour waffles is a tasty gluten-free and grain-free alternative for a delightful breakfast. Create waffle batter with coconut flour. Serve with fresh fruit and a drizzle of agave syrup.
Here's a simple recipe to guide you:

Ingredients:
- 1/2 cup coconut flour
- 1/2 teaspoon baking powder
- 1/4 teaspoon salt
- 4 large eggs
- 1/2 cup coconut milk (or any dairy-free milk)
- 2 tablespoons melted coconut oil (or any neutral oil)
- 1 tablespoon sweetener (honey, maple syrup, or your choice)
- 1 teaspoon vanilla extract

Instructions:
1. Preheat Waffle Iron:
    - Preheat your waffle iron according to its instructions.
2. Combine Dry Ingredients:
    - In a bowl, whisk together coconut flour, baking powder, and salt.
3. Mix Wet Ingredients:
    - In a separate bowl, whisk together eggs, coconut milk, melted coconut oil, sweetener, and vanilla extract.
4. Combine Wet and Dry Ingredients:

Mix thoroughly after adding the wet ingredients to the dry ingredients. Coconut flour absorbs liquid quickly, so the batter will be thicker than traditional waffle batter.

5. Let the Batter Rest:

   - Allow the batter to rest for a few minutes to let the coconut flour absorb more liquid.

6. Cook the Waffles:

   - Grease the waffle iron with a little coconut oil if needed.

   - Spoon the batter onto the hot waffle iron, spreading it out evenly.

   - Close the waffle iron and cook according to the manufacturer's instructions until the waffles are golden brown.

7. Serve Warm:

   The waffles should be served warm after being carefully taken out of the iron.

Additional Tips:

Toppings:

   - Top your coconut flour waffles with fresh fruit, shredded coconut, a drizzle of honey or maple syrup, or a dollop of dairy-free yogurt.

Texture Variation:

   - For added texture, consider incorporating ingredients like chopped nuts or shredded coconut into the batter.

Customize Flavors:
  - Experiment with flavors by adding ingredients like cinnamon, nutmeg, or a hint of citrus zest.

Make Ahead:
  - Cooked waffles can be frozen and reheated in a toaster for a quick breakfast.

Enjoy your delicious and coconut-flavored waffles as a gluten-free and delightful breakfast treat!

8. **Sweet Potato Hash**:
 Sweet potato hash is a flavorful and nutritious dish, perfect for breakfast or as a side. Dice sweet potatoes and sauté with onions, peppers, and spinach. Top with avocado slices and a sprinkle of nutritional yeast. Here's a simple recipe for you:

Ingredients:
Two medium-sized sweet potatoes, chopped and skinned
- 1 onion, diced
- 1 bell pepper, diced
- 2 tablespoons olive oil or preferred cooking oil
- 1 teaspoon smoked paprika
- 1/2 teaspoon garlic powder
- 1/2 teaspoon cumin
- Salt and pepper to taste
- For garnish, use fresh cilantro or parsley (optional).

Instructions:
1. Prep Ingredients:
   - Peel and dice the sweet potatoes into small, even cubes.
   Chop the pepper and onion.

2. Cook Sweet Potatoes:
   Heat the olive oil in a big skillet over medium heat. Cook after adding the chopped sweet potatoes for about 5-7 minutes, stirring occasionally, until they start to soften.

3. Add Onion and Bell Pepper:
   - Add the diced onion and bell pepper to the skillet with the sweet potatoes. Cook the vegetables for a further five to seven minutes, or until they are soft.

4. Season the Hash:
   - Sprinkle smoked paprika, garlic powder, cumin, salt, and pepper over the sweet potato mixture. In order to coat the vegetables with the seasonings equally, stir well.

5. Cook Until Crispy:
   - Allow the hash to cook for an additional 5-7 minutes, stirring occasionally. This will help the sweet potatoes develop a slightly crispy exterior.

6. Adjust Seasoning:
   - Taste the sweet potato hash and adjust the seasoning if necessary. To taste, increase the amount of spices, salt, or pepper.

7. Garnish and Serve:
   - Once the sweet potatoes are tender and slightly crispy, remove the skillet from heat. If desired, garnish with cilantro or fresh parsley.

8. Serve Warm:
   - Serve the sweet potato hash as a side dish, or enjoy it as a wholesome breakfast topped with a fried or poached egg.

Additional Tips:
Customize Flavors:
   - Experiment with additional spices like chili powder, cinnamon, or a dash of cayenne for extra flavor.

Protein Boost:
   - Incorporate cooked sausage, bacon, or black beans for added protein.

Make It Ahead:
   - Prepare the sweet potato hash in advance and reheat in a skillet for a quick and convenient meal.

Sweet potato hash is a versatile dish that pairs well with various proteins and makes a delicious and nutritious addition to your meals.

9. **Protein-Packed Breakfast Burrito:**
   - Fill a gluten-free tortilla with scrambled tofu, black beans, salsa, and avocado. Creating a protein-packed breakfast burrito is a delicious and satisfying way to start your day. Here's a simple recipe for you:

Ingredients:
- 1 large whole-grain or gluten-free tortilla
- 2 large eggs (or tofu for a vegan option)
- 1/4 cup washed and drained black beans
- 1/4 cup diced bell peppers
- 1/4 cup diced onions
- 1/4 cup diced tomatoes
- 1/4 cup shredded dairy-free cheese
- 1 tablespoon olive oil
- Salt and pepper to taste
- Optional toppings: Salsa, avocado slices, cilantro, hot sauce

Instructions:
1. Prepare Ingredients:
   - Dice the bell peppers, onions, and tomatoes.
   - If using eggs, beat them in a bowl. If using tofu, crumble it and set aside.

2. Cook Vegetables:
   - In a skillet over medium heat, warm the olive oil. Add diced bell peppers and onions, sautéing until softened.

3. Add Eggs or Tofu:
   - Push the veggies to the side of the skillet and pour beaten eggs or crumbled tofu into the empty space. Scramble the eggs or tofu until cooked through.

4. Add Black Beans:
   - Mix in the black beans, stirring to combine with the eggs or tofu. Heat until the beans are warmed.

5. Season:
   - Season the mixture with salt and pepper to taste.

6. Warm Tortilla:
   - In a separate skillet or directly on a gas stove flame, warm the tortilla for a few seconds on each side until pliable.

7. Assemble the Burrito:
   - Place the warm tortilla on a flat surface.
   - Spoon the egg or tofu mixture onto the center of the tortilla.

8. Add Toppings:
   - Top with diced tomatoes, dairy-free cheese, and any additional toppings you prefer.

9. Fold and Roll:
   - Fold in the sides of the tortilla and then roll it from the bottom to form a burrito.

10. Serve Warm:
   - Place the seam side down on a plate and serve immediately.

Additional Tips:
Customize Proteins:
   - Include cooked turkey sausage, bacon, or plant-based meat alternatives for additional protein.

Boost Flavor:
  - Add herbs and spices like cumin, paprika, or chili powder for extra flavor.

Meal Prep:
   - Make a batch of the filling in advance and assemble burritos on-the-go for a quick breakfast.

Adjust Spice Level:
  - Customize the heat level by adding hot sauce or adjusting the amount of spicy toppings.

This protein-packed breakfast burrito is not only a tasty morning option but also provides a balanced and energizing start to your day. Enjoy your flavorful and filling creation!

10. **Fruit Salad Parfait:**
   - Layer dairy-free yogurt with fresh fruit chunks and gluten-free granola. Creating a fruit salad parfait is a refreshing and healthy way to enjoy a delightful dessert or breakfast. Here's a simple recipe for you:

Ingredients:
- 2 cups mixed fresh fruits (berries, kiwi, pineapple, mango, etc.)
- 1 cup dairy-free yogurt (coconut, almond, soy, etc.)
- 1/2 cup gluten-free granola
- Honey or maple syrup for drizzling (optional)
- Mint leaves for garnish (optional)

Instructions:
1. Prepare Fruits:
   - Peel, cut, and wash the fruits into small pieces.

2. Layer 1 - Fruits:
   - Begin by placing a layer of mixed fruits at the bottom of each serving glass or bowl.

3. Layer 2 - Dairy-Free Yogurt:
   - Add a layer of dairy-free yogurt on top of the fruits. You can use a spoon to spread it evenly.

4. Layer 3 - Granola:
   - Sprinkle a layer of gluten-free granola over the yogurt. This adds a delightful crunch to the parfait.

5. Repeat Layers:
   - Repeat the layers until you reach the top of the glass or bowl, finishing with a final layer of fruits on top.

6. Drizzle with Sweetener:

- For a hint of sweetness, you can pour some honey or maple syrup on top if you'd like.

7. Garnish:
   - Garnish with fresh mint leaves for a burst of color and additional freshness.

8. Serve Chilled:
   - Place the fruit salad parfait in the refrigerator for at least 30 minutes before serving to allow the flavors to meld.

Additional Tips:
Customize Fruits:
   - Use a variety of fruits based on your preference and seasonal availability.

Yogurt Alternatives:
   - Experiment with different dairy-free yogurts to find your favorite flavor and consistency.

Add Nuts or Seeds:
   - Boost the nutritional content by adding a sprinkle of chopped nuts or seeds between the layers.

Make-Ahead Option:
   - Prepare the components ahead of time and assemble the parfait just before serving to maintain the granola's crunch.

Portion Control:
  - Adjust the serving size to fit your dietary needs and preferences.

This fruit salad parfait is a vibrant and customizable treat that combines the sweetness of fruits, the creaminess of yogurt, and the crunch of granola. Enjoy it as a delightful dessert or a refreshing breakfast option!

Tips for Success:
Label Reading:
  - Ensure all ingredients, including condiments, are gluten-free and dairy-free.

Homemade Nut Butter:
  - Make your nut butter using almonds, cashews, or sunflower seeds.

Egg Substitutes:
  - Use flax eggs or chia eggs as alternatives in baking.

Explore Alternative Flours:
  - Experiment with almond flour, coconut flour, or rice flour in baking.

Check Condiments:
  - Verify that sauces and condiments used are free from gluten and dairy.

A gluten-free and dairy-free breakfast can be both wholesome and flavorful, offering a variety of options to kickstart your day with energy and satisfaction.

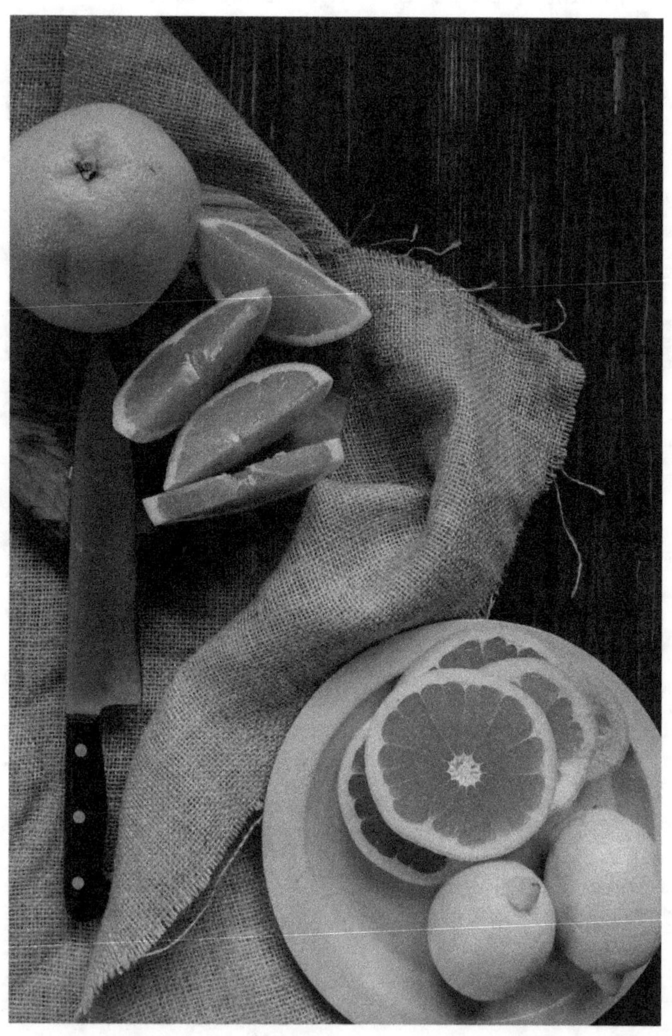

CHAPTER THREE

BRUNCH

Brunch, a delightful fusion of breakfast and lunch, has become a popular and cherished mealtime tradition. This casual and leisurely dining experience typically takes place between the typical breakfast and lunch hours, providing a perfect opportunity to savor a diverse range of culinary delights. Here's a comprehensive overview of brunch:

The Essence of Brunch:
1. Timing and Atmosphere:
   - Brunch is usually enjoyed between late morning and early afternoon, creating a relaxed and social atmosphere.
2. Diverse Menu:
   - Brunch menus often feature a diverse range of dishes, combining breakfast staples with heartier lunch options.

Brunch Components:
1. Breakfast Classics:
   - Common breakfast items like eggs (prepared in various styles), bacon, sausages, and pancakes often find a place on brunch menus.

2. Pastries and Baked Goods:
   - Croissants, muffins, scones, and pastries contribute a touch of sweetness to the brunch experience.

3. Fresh Fruits:
   - Fresh fruit salads, fruit platters, or fruit-infused beverages add a refreshing and healthy element.

4. Beverages:
   - Brunch is known for its assortment of beverages, including coffee, tea, fresh juices, and brunch-specific cocktails like mimosas or Bloody Marys.
5. Lunch Favorites:
   - Heavier dishes such as salads, sandwiches, soups, and even pasta may be part of the brunch spread.

Social and Cultural Aspects:
1. Social Gathering:
   - Brunch is often associated with socializing, making it a popular choice for gatherings with friends, family, or colleagues.
2. Weekend Tradition:
   - Many people reserve brunch for weekends, turning it into a leisurely affair to unwind and enjoy good company.
3. Special Occasions:
   - Brunch is a favored choice for celebrating special occasions such as birthdays, bridal showers, and holidays.

Contemporary Trends:
1. Health-Conscious Options:
   - Modern brunch menus often include healthier options like avocado toast, smoothie bowls, and plant-based dishes to cater to diverse dietary preferences.

2. Global Influences:
   - Fusion dishes and global influences have become prevalent, allowing brunch enthusiasts to explore a variety of flavors and cuisines.

Brunch Etiquette:
1. Reservations:
   - Popular brunch spots may require reservations, especially during peak hours.

2. Attire:
   - Brunch often has a casual dress code, creating a comfortable and laid-back atmosphere.

3. Duration:
   - Unlike hurried weekday meals, brunch is meant to be enjoyed at a leisurely pace, fostering conversation and relaxation.

Brunch is more than just a meal; it's a social experience that celebrates the best of breakfast and lunch. Whether enjoyed in a trendy cafe, a cozy neighborhood spot, or at home with loved ones, brunch continues to evolve, adapting to changing culinary trends and diverse palates. Its enduring popularity lies in its ability to offer a versatile and enjoyable dining experience for people of all ages and tastes.

Gluten-Free and Diary-Free Brunch

Embracing a gluten-free and dairy-free lifestyle doesn't mean compromising on flavor and variety, especially when it comes to brunch. There's a rich array of delicious recipes catering to these dietary preferences. Here's a comprehensive guide to gluten-free and dairy-free brunch recipes

1. **Egg Muffins with Spinach and Tomatoes:**
   - Whisk together eggs, diced tomatoes, sautéed spinach, and your favorite herbs. Pour the mixture into muffin cups and bake for convenient and portable egg muffins. Creating delicious and nutritious egg muffins with spinach and tomatoes is a straightforward process. Here's a simple recipe for you:

Ingredients:
- 6 large eggs
- 1 cup fresh spinach, chopped
- 1 cup cherry tomatoes, diced
- 1/2 cup dairy-free cheese, shredded (optional)

- Salt and pepper to taste
- Olive oil or cooking spray for greasing the muffin tin

Instructions:
1. Preheat the Oven:
   - Preheat your oven to 375°F (190°C).

2. Prepare Spinach and Tomatoes:
   - Chop fresh spinach into small pieces and dice the cherry tomatoes.

3. Sauté Spinach:
   - In a skillet over medium heat, sauté the chopped spinach until it wilts. Set aside to cool.

4. Prepare Muffin Tin:
   - Grease a muffin tin with olive oil or cooking spray to prevent sticking.

5. Whisk Eggs:
   - Using a whisk, beat the eggs thoroughly in a mixing bowl. Season with salt and pepper to taste.

6. Combine Ingredients:
   - Add the sautéed spinach, diced tomatoes, and dairy-free cheese (if using) to the whisked

eggs. For the ingredients to be distributed evenly, thoroughly mix.

7. Fill Muffin Cups:
   - Pour the egg mixture evenly into the prepared muffin cups, filling each cup about 3/4 full.

8. Bake:
   -After preheating the oven, place the muffin tray inside and bake for about 15 to 20 minutes, or until the tops of the egg muffins are set and beginning to turn brown.

9. Cool and Serve:
   - Before carefully removing the egg muffins from the muffin tin, let them cool for a few minutes. Use a butter knife or spoon to loosen the edges.

10. Serve Warm or Store:
    - Serve the egg muffins warm as a delightful brunch option. If you're making them ahead, let them cool completely before storing in an airtight container in the refrigerator.

Additional Tips:
Customize Ingredients:
  - Feel free to add other vegetables, herbs, or spices based on your preferences. Bell peppers, onions, and herbs like parsley or chives work well.

Protein Boost:

- Add cooked and crumbled bacon, sausage, or plant-based protein for an extra protein boost.

Make-Ahead Option:

- Prepare the egg muffin mixture the night before and store it in the refrigerator. In the morning, simply fill the muffin cups and bake.

Freeze for Later:

- These egg muffins freeze well. Once cooled, store them in a freezer-safe container, separated by parchment paper, and reheat when needed.

These egg muffins are not only delicious but also versatile, making them a convenient and healthy addition to your brunch or breakfast routine. Enjoy the combination of vibrant spinach and juicy tomatoes in each bite!

2. Almond Flour Banana Bread:

- Bake a moist and delicious banana bread using almond flour. Add dairy-free chocolate chips or chopped nuts for extra flavor. Baking almond flour banana bread is a delightful way to enjoy a gluten-free and moist loaf with a nutty flavor. Here's a simple recipe for you:

Ingredients:
- 3 ripe bananas, mashed
- 3 large eggs
- 1/4 cup dairy-free butter or coconut oil, melted.
- 1 teaspoon vanilla extract
- 2 cups almond flour
- 1/4 cup coconut flour
- 1 teaspoon baking soda
- 1/2 teaspoon salt
- Optional: 1/2 cup dairy-free chocolate chips, chopped nuts, or dried fruit

Instructions:
1. Preheat the Oven:
    - Preheat your oven to 350°F (175°C). Grease a standard-sized loaf pan.
2. Prepare Wet Ingredients:
    - In a large mixing bowl, mash the ripe bananas using a fork or potato masher. Add the eggs, melted coconut oil or dairy-free butter, and vanilla extract. Mix well until the ingredients are combined.
3. Combine Dry Ingredients:
    - In a separate bowl, whisk together the almond flour, coconut flour, baking soda, and salt.

4. Mix Wet and Dry Ingredients:
   - Stirring until just blended, gradually add the dry ingredients to the wet components. Take cautious not to blend too much.
5. Optional Add-ins:
   - If desired, fold in dairy-free chocolate chips, chopped nuts, or dried fruit into the batter for added texture and flavor.
6. Transfer to Pan:
   - Evenly distribute the batter into the loaf pan after greasing it.
7. Bake:
   - Bake for 45 to 55 minutes, or until a toothpick inserted in the center comes out clean, in a preheated oven.
8. Cool:
   - After letting the banana bread sit in the pan for ten to fifteen minutes, move it to a wire rack to finish cooling.
9. Slice and Serve:
   - Once completely cooled, slice the almond flour banana bread into thick slices and enjoy!

Additional Tips:
Ripe Bananas:
   - Use ripe bananas for natural sweetness and moisture in the bread.

Flour Consistency:
  - Ensure your almond flour is finely ground for a smoother texture.

Storage:
  - Store leftover banana bread in an airtight container at room temperature for a day or two. Store it in the refrigerator for extended periods of time.

Freezing:
  - Banana bread freezes well. Slice it before freezing, and you can easily grab a slice whenever you crave it.

Customize:
  - Feel free to tweak the recipe by adding your favorite mix-ins or toppings.

This almond flour banana bread recipe provides a delicious and gluten-free alternative to traditional banana bread, making it a wonderful treat for those with dietary restrictions or anyone looking for a healthier option. Enjoy the rich, nutty flavor and moist texture of this delightful banana bread!

3. **Sautéed Veggie and Tofu Scramble:**
   - Sauté diced tofu with a variety of colorful vegetables such as bell peppers, mushrooms, and spinach. Season with turmeric, cumin, and nutritional yeast for a flavorful scramble. Creating a sautéed veggie and tofu scramble is a flavorful and protein-packed breakfast or brunch option. Here's a simple recipe for you:

Ingredients:
- 1 block firm tofu, pressed and crumbled
- 2 tablespoons olive oil
- 1 bell pepper, diced
- 1 small red onion, diced
- 1 cup cherry tomatoes, halved
- 2 cups fresh spinach, chopped
- 2 cloves garlic, minced
- 1 teaspoon turmeric powder (for color)
- Salt and pepper to taste
- Add-ons: nutritional yeast for a cheesy taste; fresh herbs (parsley, chives, etc.)

Instructions:
1. Prepare Tofu:
   - Tofu should be pressed to eliminate extra water. Break it up with a fork or your hands into small pieces.

2. Sauté Vegetables:
   - Heat the olive oil in a big skillet over medium heat. Add diced bell pepper and red onion. Sauté until the vegetables are softened.

3. Add Garlic and Tomatoes:
   - In the skillet, add the minced garlic and cook for about one minute, or until fragrant. Then, add the halved cherry tomatoes and cook for an additional 2-3 minutes.

4. Incorporate Tofu:
   - Add the crumbled tofu to the skillet, mixing it with the sautéed vegetables. Cook for 5-7 minutes until the tofu starts to brown slightly.

5. Season with Turmeric and Salt:
   - Sprinkle turmeric powder over the tofu mixture for color. Season with salt and pepper to taste. Stir well to evenly distribute the spices.

6. Add Spinach:
   - Add chopped fresh spinach to the skillet. Stir and cook until the spinach wilts and is incorporated into the scramble.

7. Optional Nutritional Yeast:

- For a cheesy flavor, you can add nutritional yeast to the tofu scramble. Start with 2 tablespoons and adjust according to your taste.

8. Garnish and Serve:

- Garnish the tofu scramble with fresh herbs, such as parsley or chives. Serve warm.

Additional Tips:

Customize Vegetables:

- You can certainly change or add veggies to suit your tastes. Mushrooms, zucchini, or kale are excellent choices.

Spice it Up:

- Experiment with additional spices or herbs like cumin, paprika, or thyme to enhance the flavor.

Serve with Sides:

- Enjoy the tofu scramble on its own or serve it with avocado slices, gluten-free toast, or a side of salsa.

Protein Boost:

- For an extra protein boost, consider adding black beans or chickpeas to the scramble.

Meal Prep:

- This tofu scramble is great for meal prep. Cook a larger batch and store it in the refrigerator for quick and easy breakfasts throughout the week.

This sautéed veggie and tofu scramble is a nutritious and satisfying dish, perfect for those looking for a plant-based, gluten-free breakfast or brunch option. Enjoy the savory flavors and vibrant colors in every bite!

4. **Gluten-Free and Dairy-Free Blueberry Muffins:**
- Combine gluten-free flour, dairy-free milk, and fresh blueberries to create fluffy and flavorful blueberry muffins. Making gluten-free and dairy-free blueberry muffins is a delicious way to enjoy a classic treat without compromising dietary preferences. Here's a simple recipe for you:

Ingredients:
- 2 cups gluten-free all-purpose flour
- 1/2 cup almond flour
- 1 1/2 teaspoons baking powder
- 1/2 teaspoon baking soda
- 1/2 teaspoon salt
- 1/2 cup coconut oil, melted

- 1/2 cup maple syrup or agave nectar
- 1/2 cup soy, coconut, or almond milk substituted for dairy

- 2 flax eggs (2 tablespoons flaxseed meal + 6 tablespoons water)
- 1 teaspoon vanilla extract
- 1/2 cup blueberries, either frozen or fresh

Instructions:
1. Preheat the Oven:
   - Preheat your oven to 350°F (175°C). Use paper liners to line a muffin tray.

2. Prepare Flax Eggs:
   - In a small bowl, mix 2 tablespoons of flaxseed meal with 6 tablespoons of water. Let it sit for about 5 minutes until it forms a gel-like consistency.

3. Combine Dry Ingredients:
   - In a large mixing bowl, whisk together the gluten-free all-purpose flour, almond flour, baking powder, baking soda, and salt.

4. Mix Wet Ingredients:
   - In a separate bowl, combine the melted coconut oil, maple syrup or agave nectar,

dairy-free milk, flax eggs, and vanilla extract. Mix well.

5. Combine Wet and Dry Ingredients:
   - Mixing until just mixed, pour the wet components into the dry ingredients. Take care not to mix too much.

6. Add Blueberries:
   - Once the blueberries are properly mixed into the batter, gently fold them in.

7. Fill Muffin Cups:
   - Pour the mixture into the muffin tins, filling each to about two thirds of the way.

8. Bake:
   - A toothpick put into the center of a muffin should come out clean after 20 to 25 minutes of baking in a preheated oven.

9. Cool:
   - Allow the blueberry muffins to cool in the muffin tin for 5 minutes, then transfer them to a wire rack to cool completely.

10. Enjoy:

- Once cooled, these gluten-free and dairy-free blueberry muffins are ready to be enjoyed!

Additional Tips:

Frozen Blueberries:

- If using frozen blueberries, toss them in a little gluten-free flour before adding to the batter to prevent them from sinking to the bottom.

Storage:

- Leftover muffins can be kept for a day or two at room temperature in an airtight container. For longer storage, keep them in the refrigerator.

Freezing:

- These muffins freeze well. Place them in a zip-top bag, and they'll be ready to grab whenever you want a quick and tasty snack.

Customization:

- Feel free to add a streusel topping, chopped nuts, or a sprinkle of cinnamon sugar for extra flavor and texture.

These gluten-free and dairy-free blueberry muffins are a delightful treat suitable for a variety of dietary needs. Enjoy the burst of blueberry goodness in a moist and tender muffin!

5. **Cauliflower Hash Browns**:

   - Grate cauliflower and mix it with gluten-free flour, seasonings, and flaxseed meal. Shape into patties and pan-fry until golden brown for a low-carb alternative to hash browns. Making cauliflower hash browns is a flavorful and low-carb alternative to traditional potato hash browns. Here's a simple recipe for you:

Ingredients:
- 1 medium-sized cauliflower head, grated
- 2 flax eggs (2 tablespoons flaxseed meal + 6 tablespoons water)
- 1/4 cup gluten-free all-purpose flour
- 1/4 cup nutritional yeast (optional, for a cheesy flavor)
- 1 teaspoon garlic powder
- 1/2 teaspoon onion powder
- Salt and pepper to taste
- Cooking oil for frying

Instructions:
1. Prepare Flax Eggs:
   - In a small bowl, mix 2 tablespoons of flaxseed meal with 6 tablespoons of water. Allow it to sit for about 5 minutes until it forms a gel-like consistency.

2. Grate Cauliflower:
   - Use a food processor or a box grater to finely chop the cauliflower. You can also use the pulse function of the food processor to achieve a rice-like consistency.

3. Squeeze Out Moisture:
   - Place the grated cauliflower in a clean kitchen towel or cheesecloth and squeeze out excess moisture. This step is crucial to achieving crispy hash browns.

4. Combine Ingredients:
   - In a large mixing bowl, combine the grated cauliflower, flax eggs, gluten-free all-purpose flour, nutritional yeast (if using), garlic powder, onion powder, salt, and pepper. Mix until well combined.

5. Form Patties:
   - Take a portion of the mixture and shape it into a patty with your hands. The mixture should hold together well.

6. Heat Cooking Oil:
   - In a skillet over medium heat, preheat cooking oil. Ensure the oil is hot before adding the hash browns to achieve a crispy exterior.

7. Cook Hash Browns:
   - Carefully place the cauliflower hash brown patties in the hot skillet. Cook for 3-4 minutes on each side or until golden brown and crisp.

8. Drain Excess Oil:
   - Once cooked, transfer the hash browns to a plate lined with paper towels to drain any excess oil.

9. Repeat:
   - Continue with the remaining cauliflower mixture, adjusting the skillet's oil level as necessary.

10. Serve Warm:
   - Serve the cauliflower hash browns warm as a delicious and low-carb alternative to traditional hash browns.

Additional Tips:
Spice it Up:
  - Customize the flavor by adding your favorite spices or herbs, such as paprika, cayenne pepper, or chopped fresh herbs.

Dipping Sauce:
  - Pair the cauliflower hash browns with your favorite dairy-free dipping sauce, like vegan aioli or ketchup.

Oven-Baked Option:
  - For a healthier option, you can bake the cauliflower hash browns in the oven. Place them on a lined baking sheet and bake at 400°F (200°C) for about 20-25 minutes, flipping halfway through.

Freezing:
  - Freeze any leftover hash browns in a single layer on a baking sheet, then transfer to a freezer bag. Reheat in the oven or toaster oven for a quick and convenient snack.

These cauliflower hash browns are a tasty and nutritious alternative, providing a satisfying crunch without the traditional starch. Enjoy them as a side dish or as part of a hearty breakfast or brunch!

6. Coconut Milk Chia Seed Pancakes:

- Blend coconut milk, chia seeds, and gluten-free flour to make a unique pancake batter. Serve with a tropical fruit compote for added freshness. Creating coconut milk chia seed pancakes is a delightful way to enjoy a gluten-free and dairy-free breakfast. Here's a simple recipe for you:

Ingredients:
- 1 cup gluten-free all-purpose flour
- 1 tablespoon chia seeds
- 1 teaspoon baking powder
- 1/4 teaspoon salt
- 1 cup coconut milk
- 2 tablespoons coconut oil, melted
- 2 tablespoons maple syrup or agave nectar
- 1 teaspoon vanilla extract
- Additional coconut oil for greasing the skillet

Instructions:
1. Prepare Chia Seeds:

- In a small bowl, mix the chia seeds with 3 tablespoons of water. Let it sit for about 5 minutes until it forms a gel-like consistency. This will act as an egg substitute.

2. Combine Dry Ingredients:

   - In a large mixing bowl, whisk together the gluten-free all-purpose flour, baking powder, and salt.

3. Mix Wet Ingredients:

   - In another bowl, combine the coconut milk, melted coconut oil, maple syrup or agave nectar, vanilla extract, and the chia seed gel. Mix well.

4. Combine Wet and Dry Ingredients:

   - Mixing until just mixed, pour the wet components into the dry ingredients. Take care not to overmix; some lumps are acceptable.

5. Let the Batter Rest:

   - Give the batter ten to fifteen minutes to rest. This allows the chia seeds to further absorb liquid and the batter to thicken.

6. Preheat the Skillet:

   - Heat a griddle or nonstick skillet to medium. Add a small amount of coconut oil to grease the surface.

7. Cook Pancakes:

   - Pour 1/4 cup of batter for each pancake onto the hot skillet. Cook until bubbles form on the surface and the edges start to set, then flip and cook the other side until golden brown.

8. Repeat:

   - Proceed with the leftover batter, adjusting the amount of coconut oil in the skillet as necessary.

9. Serve Warm:

   - Serve the coconut milk chia seed pancakes warm with your favorite toppings, such as fresh fruit, dairy-free yogurt, or maple syrup.

Additional Tips:
Coconut Flakes:

   - For an extra coconut flavor and texture, you can add shredded coconut or coconut flakes to the pancake batter.

Spice it Up:

   - Enhance the flavor with a pinch of cinnamon or nutmeg in the batter.

Dairy-Free Toppings:

   - Top your pancakes with dairy-free alternatives like coconut whipped cream or a drizzle of chocolate sauce.

Make a Batch:
  - This recipe can easily be doubled or halved based on your needs. Pancakes leftovers can be reheated in the refrigerator.

These coconut milk chia seed pancakes offer a delightful tropical twist to your morning routine. Enjoy the combination of coconut and chia seeds in a stack

of fluffy, gluten-free goodness. Whether you're following a specific dietary lifestyle or just craving a unique pancake experience, these coconut milk chia seed pancakes are sure to be a hit at your breakfast table.

7. Dairy-Free Frittata with Veggies:

  - Whisk together eggs and dairy-free milk. Pour the mixture over sautéed vegetables in an oven-safe skillet and bake until set for a delicious dairy-free frittata. Making a dairy-free frittata with veggies is a flavorful and versatile option for a satisfying breakfast or brunch. Here's a simple recipe for you:

Ingredients:
- 1 tablespoon olive oil
- 1 small onion, diced
- 2 bell peppers (any color), diced

- 1 zucchini, diced
- 1 cup cherry tomatoes, halved
- 8 large eggs
- 1/4 cup dairy-free milk (almond, coconut, or soy)
- Salt and pepper to taste
- 1 teaspoon dried herbs (such as thyme, oregano, or rosemary)
- Fresh herbs for garnish (optional)

Instructions:
1. Preheat the Oven:
   - Preheat your oven to 375°F (190°C).
2. Sauté Vegetables:
   - In an oven-safe skillet, heat olive oil over medium heat. Add diced onion and sauté until translucent. Add bell peppers and zucchini, cooking until softened. Finally, add halved cherry tomatoes and cook for an additional 2 minutes.
3. Whisk Eggs and Milk:
   - In a mixing bowl, whisk together eggs, dairy-free milk, salt, pepper, and dried herbs until well combined.

4. Combine Eggs and Veggies:
   - Over the skillet's sautéed veggies, pour the egg mixture. Gently stir to ensure even distribution.

5. Cook on the Stovetop:
   - Allow the frittata to cook on the stovetop for 2-3 minutes, letting the edges set.

6. Transfer to the Oven:
   - Transfer the skillet to the preheated oven and bake for 15-20 minutes or until the frittata is set in the center and the top is lightly golden.

7. Broil (Optional):
   - If you want a golden top, you can broil the frittata for an additional 1-2 minutes, but keep a close eye to prevent burning.

8. Garnish and Serve:
   - Remove the frittata from the oven. Garnish with fresh herbs if desired. Let it cool down a little before slicing.

9. Serve Warm:
   - Serve the dairy-free frittata warm, either directly from the skillet or by transferring it to a serving platter.

Additional Tips:
Vegetable Variations:

- Feel free to customize the frittata with your favorite vegetables such as spinach, mushrooms, or asparagus.

Cheesy Flavor (Optional):
- If you miss the cheesy flavor, add a sprinkle of nutritional yeast or your favorite dairy-free cheese to the egg mixture.

Protein Boost:
- Enhance the protein content by adding cooked and crumbled tofu or chickpeas to the egg mixture.

Make-Ahead:
- This dairy-free frittata is excellent for meal prep. You can make it ahead of time and refrigerate it, reheating slices as needed.

This dairy-free frittata is a versatile dish that allows you to get creative with your favorite veggies and flavorings. Enjoy a slice for breakfast, brunch, or even a quick and satisfying dinner.

8. **Gluten-Free Zucchini Bread**:
- Utilize gluten-free flour and shredded zucchini to bake a moist and flavorful zucchini bread. Add cinnamon and nutmeg for extra

warmth. Creating a delicious gluten-free zucchini bread is a wonderful way to enjoy a moist and flavorful treat. Here's a simple recipe for you:

Ingredients:
- About two medium-sized zucchini, or two cups of shredded zucchini
- 3 large eggs
- 1/2 cup melted coconut oil or vegetable oil
- 1/2 cup unsweetened applesauce
- One cup of coconut sugar or granulated sugar.
- 2 teaspoons vanilla extract
- 2 cups gluten-free all-purpose flour
- 1 teaspoon baking powder
- 1/2 teaspoon baking soda
- 1/2 teaspoon salt
- 1 teaspoon ground cinnamon
- 1/2 teaspoon ground nutmeg (optional)
- Half a cup of chocolate chips or chopped almonds (optional).

Instructions:
1. Preheat the Oven:
    - Preheat your oven to 350°F (175°C). Grease and flour a loaf pan that is standard size.

2. Grate Zucchini:
   - Using a box grater, finely shred the zucchini. Place the grated zucchini in a clean kitchen towel and squeeze out excess moisture.

3. Prepare Wet Ingredients:
   - In a large mixing bowl, whisk together the eggs, melted coconut oil or vegetable oil, applesauce, sugar, and vanilla extract.

4. Combine Dry Ingredients:
   - In a separate bowl, whisk together the gluten-free all-purpose flour, baking powder, baking soda, salt, ground cinnamon, and ground nutmeg (if using).

5. Mix Batter:
   - Mixing until just mixed, add the dry ingredients to the wet ones. Don't mix too much. The batter will be thick.

6. Fold in Zucchini and Optional Add-ins:
   - Once the zucchini has been grated, gently mix it into the batter until it is uniformly distributed. Add chocolate chips or chopped nuts, if preferred.

7. Fill the Loaf Pan:
   - Evenly distribute the batter throughout the loaf pan after pouring it in.

8. Bake:
   - Bake for 50–60 minutes, or until a toothpick inserted in the center comes out clean or contains a few wet crumbs, depending on the temperature setting.

9. Cool:
   - Allow the zucchini bread to cool in the pan for about 10 minutes before transferring it to a wire rack to cool completely.

10. Slice and Serve:
    - Slice the gluten-free zucchini bread and enjoy after it has cooled!

Additional Tips:
Gluten-Free Flour:
   - Choose a high-quality gluten-free all-purpose flour blend for the best texture. You can find pre-made blends at most grocery stores.

Sugar Alternatives:
  - If you prefer a less sweet option, you can use coconut sugar or reduce the amount of sugar in the recipe.

Nut-Free Option:
  - Omit nuts if you have allergies or replace them with seeds such as pumpkin or sunflower seeds.

Storage:
  - Store leftover zucchini bread in an airtight container at room temperature for a day or two. Store it in the refrigerator for extended periods of time.

Freezing:
  - Zucchini bread freezes well. To facilitate portioning, slice it before freezing.

Enjoy the delightful flavors of this gluten-free zucchini bread, perfect for breakfast, snacking, or a sweet treat any time of the day!

9. **Sweet Potato and Kale Breakfast Casserole**:
   - Layer sliced sweet potatoes, kale, and dairy-free cheese in a baking dish. Pour a mixture of whisked eggs and dairy-free milk

over the layers and bake until golden brown. Creating a sweet potato and kale breakfast casserole is a nutritious and flavorful option for a satisfying morning meal. Here's a simple recipe for you:

Ingredients:
- 2 medium-sized sweet potatoes, peeled and grated
- 2 cups kale, chopped
- 1 small onion, finely chopped
- 1 red bell pepper, diced
- 8 large eggs
- 1 cup dairy-free milk (almond, coconut, or soy)
- 1 teaspoon garlic powder
- 1 teaspoon smoked paprika
- Salt and pepper to taste
- Olive oil for greasing the baking dish
- Optional: 1 cup dairy-free cheese, shredded

Instructions:
1. Preheat the Oven:
    - Preheat your oven to 375°F (190°C). Grease a baking dish with olive oil.
2. Prepare Sweet Potatoes:
    - Using a box grater, peel and shred the sweet potatoes. Squeeze out excess moisture using a clean kitchen towel.

3. Sauté Vegetables:

   - Heat the olive oil in a pan over medium heat. Add chopped onion and sauté until translucent. Add diced red bell pepper and continue cooking for another 2-3 minutes. Finally, add chopped kale and cook until wilted. Remove from heat.

4. Whisk Eggs and Milk:

   - In a large mixing bowl, whisk together eggs, dairy-free milk, garlic powder, smoked paprika, salt, and pepper.

5. Combine Ingredients:

   - Add the grated sweet potatoes, sautéed vegetables, and shredded dairy-free cheese (if using) to the egg mixture. Mix well to combine.

6. Transfer to Baking Dish

   - Evenly spread the ingredients as you pour it onto the baking dish that has been oiled.

7. Bake:

   - Bake for 30 to 35 minutes, or until the center is set and the sides are golden brown.

8. Cool and Slice:
   - Allow the breakfast casserole to cool for a few minutes before slicing it into squares or wedges.

9. Serve Warm:
   - Serve the sweet potato and kale breakfast casserole warm. It can be enjoyed on its own or with your favorite hot sauce or salsa.

Additional Tips:
Customize Vegetables:
   - You can certainly change or add veggies to suit your tastes. In this casserole, spinach, mushrooms, or tomatoes are good options.

Protein Boost:
   - Add cooked and crumbled sausage, tofu, or chickpeas for an extra protein boost.

Fresh Herbs:
   - Enhance the flavor by adding fresh herbs like parsley, chives, or cilantro.

Make-Ahead Option:
   -The night before, make the casserole, cover it, and put it in the fridge. Bake it in the morning for a quick and convenient breakfast.

This sweet potato and kale breakfast casserole is a hearty and wholesome dish that provides a balance of flavors and nutrients. Enjoy a tasty and filling breakfast to kickstart your day!

10. **Dairy-Free Spinach and Mushroom Quiche:**

- Create a gluten-free crust using almond flour or gluten-free oats. Fill it with a mixture of sautéed spinach, mushrooms, and a dairy-free custard made from coconut or almond milk. Making a dairy-free spinach and mushroom quiche is a flavorful and satisfying dish for breakfast or brunch. Here's a simple recipe for you:

Ingredients:
For the Crust:
- 1 1/4 cups gluten-free all-purpose flour
- 1/2 cup dairy-free butter, chilled and cubed
- 3-4 tablespoons ice-cold water

For the Filling:
- 1 tablespoon olive oil
- 1 small onion, finely chopped
- 2 cups mushrooms, sliced
- 3 cups fresh spinach, chopped
- 1 clove garlic, minced
- 8 large eggs

- 1 cup dairy-free milk (almond, coconut, or soy)
- Salt and pepper to taste
- 1/2 teaspoon dried thyme (optional)
- 1/2 cup dairy-free cheese, shredded (optional)

Instructions:
For the Crust:
1. Prepare the Crust:
    - In a food processor, combine the gluten-free all-purpose flour and chilled dairy-free butter. Pulse until the mixture resembles coarse crumbs. One spoonful at a time, add the ice-cold water, and pulse until the dough comes together.

2. Form the Crust:
   - Gather the dough into a ball, wrap it in plastic wrap, and refrigerate for at least 30 minutes.

3. Roll Out the Dough:
   - Preheat your oven to 375°F (190°C). On a lightly floured surface, roll out the chilled dough to fit a pie dish. Transfer the dough to the dish, pressing it gently against the sides. Trim any excess dough.

4. Pre-Bake the Crust:

- Pie weights or dried beans can be used to fill the parchment paper-lined crust. Pre-bake the crust for 15 minutes. Remove the weights and parchment paper, then bake for an additional 5 minutes until lightly golden.

For the Filling:
5. Sauté Vegetables:

- Heat the olive oil in a pan over medium heat. Sauté the chopped onion until it turns transparent. Sliced mushrooms should be added and cooked until their moisture is released. Add the chopped spinach and minced garlic, and heat until the spinach wilts. Take it off the fire and let it to cool a little.

6. Prepare Egg Mixture:

- In a bowl, whisk together eggs, dairy-free milk, salt, pepper, and dried thyme if using.

7. Assemble the Quiche:

- Spread the sautéed vegetable mixture evenly over the pre-baked crust. Pour the egg mixture over the vegetables. Optionally, sprinkle dairy-free cheese on top.

8. Bake:
   - Bake in the preheated oven for 30-35 minutes or until the quiche is set and golden brown on top.

9. Cool and Serve:
   - Allow the dairy-free spinach and mushroom quiche to cool for a few minutes before slicing. Serve warm.

Additional Tips:
Dairy-Free Cheese:
   - Choose a dairy-free cheese that melts well for added flavor. It's also optional to leave it out.

Crust Variation:
   - If you prefer a crustless quiche, you can skip the crust and pour the filling directly into a greased pie dish.

Herb Options:
   - Experiment with different herbs like rosemary, thyme, or basil to enhance the flavor of the quiche.

Make-Ahead:

- Prepare the quiche a day ahead, refrigerate it overnight, and bake it in the morning for a quick breakfast.

This dairy-free spinach and mushroom quiche is a delicious and wholesome option that caters to various dietary preferences. Enjoy the rich and savory flavors in every bite!

11. **Chickpea Flour Pancakes (Socca):**

- Mix chickpea flour with water and seasonings to create a batter. Cook like pancakes and serve with fresh herbs and a squeeze of lemon for a unique twist. Creating chickpea flour pancakes, also known as socca, is a simple and gluten-free alternative to traditional pancakes. Here's a straightforward recipe for you:

Ingredients:

- 1 cup chickpea flour
- 1 cup water
- 2 tablespoons olive oil
- 1/2 teaspoon salt
- 1/4 teaspoon black pepper (optional)
- 1/2 teaspoon cumin (optional)
- chopped herbs (optional: add parsley or cilantro)

Instructions:
1. Prepare the Batter:

   - In a mixing bowl, whisk together chickpea flour, water, olive oil, salt, and any optional ingredients like black pepper, cumin, or chopped herbs. Ensure a smooth and lump-free batter.

2. Rest the Batter:

   - Let the batter rest for at least 30 minutes, allowing the chickpea flour to fully absorb the water.

3. Preheat the Oven:

   - Preheat your oven broiler on high. Place an oven-proof skillet (preferably cast iron) in the oven to heat.
4. Grease the Skillet:

   - Carefully remove the hot skillet from the oven. Add a bit of olive oil to coat the bottom evenly.

5. Pour and Swirl the Batter:

   - Pour the batter into the hot skillet, swirling it to ensure an even distribution.

6. Broil:

   - Place the skillet under the broiler for 5-7 minutes or until the socca is set, golden brown around the edges, and has a few darker spots on top.

7. Cool and Slice:
   - Allow the chickpea flour pancake to cool for a few minutes. It will firm up as it cools. Slice it into wedges or squares.

8. Serve Warm:
   - Serve the socca warm as is or with your favorite toppings. It can be enjoyed with dips, spreads, or as a side dish.

Additional Tips:
Topping Ideas:
   - Top the socca with ingredients like olive tapenade, hummus, fresh herbs, or a drizzle of tahini for added flavor.

Spice Variation:
   - Customize the flavor by adding spices like smoked paprika, turmeric, or chili powder to the batter.

Herb Choices:
   - Experiment with different herbs to enhance the taste. Fresh parsley, cilantro, or chives work well.

Thickness Adjustments:

- Thinner socca will be more like a crepe, while a thicker batter will result in a heartier pancake. The amount of water can be adjusted to get the appropriate thickness.

Cooking Options:

- While broiling is a common method, you can also cook socca on the stovetop. Pour the batter into a hot, oiled skillet and cook each side until set.

Chickpea flour pancakes are not only delicious but also a great source of protein. Whether enjoyed on their own or paired with various toppings, socca provides a versatile and gluten-free alternative for pancake lovers.

Tips for Gluten-Free and Dairy-Free Brunch Cooking:
1. Dairy-Free Milk Alternatives:

- Experiment with various dairy-free milk alternatives such as almond, coconut, soy, or oat milk to find the one that complements each dish.

2. Flax or Chia Eggs:

- Use flaxseed meal or chia seeds mixed with water as egg substitutes in baking.

3. Nuts and Seeds:

   - Incorporate nuts and seeds like almonds, walnuts, chia seeds, and flaxseeds for added texture, flavor, and nutrition.

4. Fresh Herbs:

   - Elevate your dishes with fresh herbs like parsley, cilantro, basil, or dill for a burst of freshness.

5. Gluten-Free Whole Grains:

   - Explore gluten-free whole grains like quinoa, brown rice, and buckwheat for a nutrient-rich base to your brunch recipes.

These gluten-free and dairy-free brunch recipes offer a range of flavors and textures, ensuring a satisfying and enjoyable meal for everyone at the table. Whether you're catering to dietary restrictions or simply looking for tasty and wholesome options, these recipes have you covered.

CHAPTER FOUR

Lunch

Adopting a gluten-free and dairy-free lifestyle can open up a world of delicious and nutritious lunch options. Here's a comprehensive guide to crafting satisfying meals without gluten and dairy:

Base Ingredients:
1. Gluten-Free Grains:
   - Quinoa, rice, millet, buckwheat, and amaranth are excellent choices.

2. Proteins:
   - Lean meats, poultry, fish, tofu, tempeh, legumes (chickpeas, lentils), and beans.

3. Vegetables:
   - A rainbow of fresh, seasonal veggies provides essential nutrients.

4. Healthy Fats:
   - Avocado, olive oil, coconut oil, and nuts are great sources.

Recipe Ideas:
1. Gluten-Free and Dairy-Free Buddha Bowl:
   - Combine quinoa, roasted veggies, avocado slices, and your choice of protein. Drizzle with a tahini or olive oil-based dressing.

2. Grilled Chicken and Veggie Skewers:
   - Skewer marinated chicken with colorful veggies and grill. Serve with a side of quinoa or rice.

3. Chickpea and Avocado Salad:
   - Mix chickpeas, diced avocado, cherry tomatoes, cucumber, and red onion. Add lemon juice, olive oil, salt, and pepper to the dressing.
4. Salmon and Asparagus Foil Packets:
   - Place salmon fillets and asparagus on a foil sheet. Season and drizzle with lemon juice and olive oil. Close and cook.

5. Mexican Quinoa Bowl:
   - Layer cooked quinoa with black beans, corn, diced tomatoes, and grilled chicken. Top with salsa and guacamole.

6. Lentil and Vegetable Curry:
   - Simmer lentils, sweet potatoes, and veggies in coconut milk and curry spices. Serve over rice or gluten-free noodles.

7. Turkey Lettuce Wraps:
   - Sauté ground turkey with taco seasoning. Spoon into lettuce leaves and top with salsa and avocado.

8. Veggie Stir-Fry with Tofu:
   - Stir-fry a colorful mix of veggies with tofu in gluten-free tamari or soy sauce. Serve over rice.

9. Quinoa and Chickpea Stuffed Peppers:
   - Mix cooked quinoa and chickpeas with diced veggies. Bake bell peppers stuffed until they are soft.

10. Mediterranean Salad with Grilled Chicken:
   - Combine mixed greens, olives, cherry tomatoes, cucumber, and grilled chicken. Dress with olive oil and lemon vinaigrette.

Tips for Gluten-Free and Dairy-Free Lunches:
1. Dairy-Free Substitutes:
   - Experiment with almond milk, coconut milk, or soy-based dairy alternatives in recipes.

2. Gluten-Free Condiments:
   - Opt for gluten-free soy sauce, tamari, and Worcestershire sauce.

3. Read Labels:
   - Be vigilant about hidden gluten or dairy in processed foods. Choose products labeled gluten-free and dairy-free.

4. Gluten-Free Flours:
   - Explore alternative flours like almond flour, coconut flour, or rice flour for baking or thickening.

5. Fresh and Whole Foods:
   - Focus on whole, fresh ingredients to ensure a balanced and nutrient-rich meal.

6. Season with Herbs and Spices:
   - Enhance flavors with fresh herbs, spices, and citrus rather than relying on dairy for richness.

7. Meal Prep:
   - Plan and prep your lunches for the week to ensure you have satisfying options readily available.

By incorporating these base ingredients and recipe ideas, you can enjoy a diverse and delicious array of gluten-free and dairy-free lunches. The key is to experiment with flavors, embrace fresh produce, and discover the joy of creating wholesome meals that align with your dietary preferences.
 Here's a collection of comprehensive lunch recipes that cater to these dietary preferences:

1. Quinoa Salad with Roasted Vegetables:
Ingredients:
- Cooked quinoa
- Different roasted veggies (bell peppers, zucchini, cherry tomatoes)
- Fresh spinach or arugula
- For the dressing, mix olive oil, lemon juice, salt, and pepper.

Instructions:
1. Combine quinoa, roasted vegetables, and fresh greens in a bowl.

2. Whisk together olive oil, lemon juice, salt, and pepper for a light dressing.
3. Serve the salad after tossing it with the dressing.

2. **Grilled Chicken Lettuce Wraps**:
Ingredients:
- Grilled chicken strips
- Lettuce leaves (butter lettuce works well)
- Sliced avocado
- Salsa or pico de gallo

Instructions:
1. Place grilled chicken strips and avocado slices onto lettuce leaves.
2. Top with salsa or pico de gallo.
3. Wrap and secure with toothpicks for a handheld lunch.

3. **Eggplant and Tomato Stacks**:
Ingredients:
- Sliced eggplant
- Sliced tomatoes
- Dairy-free pesto
- Fresh basil leaves

Instructions:
1. Grill or bake eggplant slices until tender.
2. Assemble stacks by layering eggplant, tomato, and basil.
3. Drizzle with dairy-free pesto before serving.

4. **Salmon and Quinoa Bowl**:
Ingredients:
- Grilled or baked salmon fillets
- Cooked quinoa
- Steamed broccoli
- Avocado slices
- Lemon-tahini dressing

Instructions:
1. Arrange quinoa, salmon, steamed broccoli, and avocado in a bowl.
2. Drizzle with a dressing made from lemon juice and tahini.

5. **Chickpea and Vegetable Stir-Fry:**
Ingredients:
- Chickpeas
- Mixed stir-fry vegetables (bell peppers, broccoli, snap peas)
- Gluten-free tamari or soy sauce
- Sesame oil

Instructions:
1. Sauté chickpeas and vegetables in sesame oil.
2. Add gluten-free tamari for flavor.
3. Serve over rice or gluten-free noodles.

6. **Turkey and Avocado Lettuce Cups:**
Ingredients:
- Ground turkey, cooked with taco seasoning
- Lettuce leaves
- Diced tomatoes

- Guacamole

Instructions:
1. Spoon seasoned ground turkey into lettuce cups.
2. Top with diced tomatoes and a dollop of guacamole.

7. **Sweet Potato and Lentil Curry**:
Ingredients:
- Sweet potatoes, diced
- Cooked lentils
- Coconut milk
- Curry spices (turmeric, cumin, coriander)
- Fresh cilantro for garnish

Instructions:
1. Simmer sweet potatoes, lentils, and spices in coconut milk.
2. Garnish with fresh cilantro before serving.

Tips for Gluten-Free and Dairy-Free Lunches:
Explore Gluten-Free Grains: Incorporate grains like quinoa, rice, and millet into your meals.

Dairy-Free Substitutes: Use plant-based alternatives like almond milk, coconut milk, or soy milk in recipes.

Read Labels: Be vigilant about checking labels for hidden gluten or dairy ingredients.

Fresh Ingredients: Focus on fresh vegetables, fruits, lean proteins, and gluten-free grains for a balanced meal.

These lunch recipes offer a diverse and satisfying range of flavors, ensuring that a gluten-free and dairy-free lifestyle can be both enjoyable and nutritious.

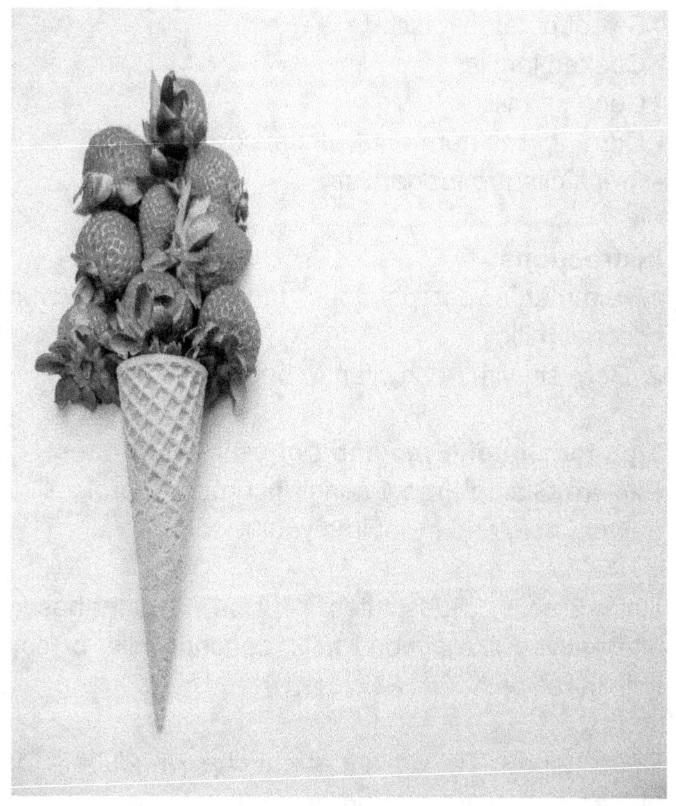

CHAPTER FIVE

Dinner

Embracing a gluten-free and dairy-free dinner routine opens up a world of flavorful and nutritious options. Here's a comprehensive guide to crafting satisfying dinners without gluten and dairy:

Base Ingredients:
1. Proteins:
     - Choose lean meats (chicken, turkey, fish), plant-based proteins (tofu, tempeh, legumes), and alternative protein sources (quinoa, buckwheat).

2. Gluten-Free Grains:
   - Utilize grains like rice, quinoa, millet, amaranth, and gluten-free pasta.

3. Vegetables:
     - Incorporate a colorful array of vegetables to ensure a variety of nutrients.

4. Healthy Fats:
   - Include avocado, olive oil, coconut oil, nuts, and seeds for essential fats.

Recipe Ideas:
1. Grilled Salmon with Lemon Herb Quinoa:

- Grill salmon fillets and serve over a bed of quinoa seasoned with lemon, fresh herbs, and olive oil.

2. Vegetable Stir-Fry with Tofu:
   - Stir-fry a mix of colorful veggies and tofu in gluten-free tamari or soy sauce. Serve over rice or gluten-free noodles.

3. Chicken and Vegetable Curry:
   - Simmer chicken and a variety of vegetables in a dairy-free coconut milk-based curry sauce. Serve over rice.

4. Mushroom and Spinach Stuffed Chicken Breasts:
   - Stuff chicken breasts with a blend of garlic, spinach, and sautéed mushrooms. Bake the chicken until it's thoroughly done.

5. Gluten-Free Spaghetti Bolognese:
   - Replace traditional pasta with gluten-free spaghetti. Prepare a hearty Bolognese sauce with ground turkey, tomatoes, and herbs.

6. Chickpea and Vegetable Tagine:
   - Create a Moroccan-inspired tagine with chickpeas, carrots, bell peppers, and tomatoes. Season with cumin, coriander, and cinnamon.

7. Cauliflower Fried Rice with Shrimp:
   - Pulse cauliflower in a food processor to create rice-sized grains. Stir-fry with shrimp, vegetables, and gluten-free soy sauce.

8. Quinoa-Stuffed Bell Peppers:
   - Mix cooked quinoa with black beans, corn, and spices. Stuff bell peppers and bake until peppers are tender.

9. Baked Chicken with Sweet Potato Wedges:
   - Coat chicken with a gluten-free spice rub and bake alongside sweet potato wedges.

10. Eggplant and Zucchini Lasagna:
   - Replace traditional pasta with layers of thinly sliced eggplant and zucchini. Fill with dairy-free ricotta and marinara sauce.

Tips for Gluten-Free and Dairy-Free Dinners:
1. Dairy-Free Substitutes:
   - Experiment with coconut milk, almond milk, or cashew cream in place of dairy milk or cream.

2. Gluten-Free Baking:
   - Use gluten-free flours (almond, coconut, rice) in place of wheat flour for baking.

3. Read Labels:
   - Be cautious of hidden gluten or dairy in processed foods. Opt for products clearly labeled gluten-free and dairy-free.

4. Fresh Herbs and Spices:
   - Elevate flavors with fresh herbs, spices, and citrus to compensate for the absence of dairy.

5. Gluten-Free Sauces:
   - Choose gluten-free soy sauce, tamari, and other condiments to avoid gluten-containing additives.

6. Nutritional Yeast:
   - Incorporate nutritional yeast for a cheesy flavor without dairy.

7. Meal Planning:
   - Plan your dinners ahead of time to ensure you have the necessary gluten-free and dairy-free ingredients on hand.

By incorporating these base ingredients and recipe ideas, you can enjoy a diverse and flavorful range of gluten-free and dairy-free dinners. The key is to experiment, explore new ingredients, and savor the richness of whole, fresh foods.

Here's a comprehensive list of 20 dinner recipes that are both gluten-free and dairy-free:

1. Grilled Lemon Herb Chicken with Quinoa:
   - Marinate chicken in lemon, garlic, and herbs. Grill and serve over a bed of seasoned quinoa.

2. Shrimp and Broccoli Stir-Fry with Rice Noodles:
   - Quickly stir-fry shrimp, broccoli, and rice noodles in a gluten-free soy sauce.

3. Mango Salsa Chicken with Cauliflower Rice:
   - Top grilled chicken with fresh mango salsa and serve over cauliflower rice.

4. Baked Lemon Garlic Salmon with Roasted Vegetables:
   - Bake salmon fillets with a lemon garlic marinade. Roast vegetables on the side.

5. Vegetable Curry with Chickpeas and Basmati Rice:
   - Create a flavorful vegetable curry using coconut milk, chickpeas, and serve over basmati rice.

6. Turkey and Quinoa Stuffed Bell Peppers:
   - Mix ground turkey, quinoa, black beans, and spices to stuff bell peppers. Bake until tender.

7. Gluten-Free Spaghetti with Tomato Basil Sauce and Meatballs:
   - Use gluten-free spaghetti with a homemade tomato basil sauce and meatballs.

8. Cauliflower Alfredo Pasta with Grilled Chicken:
   - Create a dairy-free Alfredo sauce using cauliflower. Toss with gluten-free pasta and grilled chicken.

9. Sesame Ginger Tofu Stir-Fry with Brown Rice:
   - Sauté tofu with sesame ginger sauce and colorful vegetables. Serve over brown rice.

10. Lemon Dill Baked Cod with Sweet Potato Mash:
   - Bake cod with a lemon dill marinade. Serve with mashed sweet potatoes.

11. Quinoa and Black Bean Burrito Bowls:
   - Assemble bowls with quinoa, black beans, corn, avocado, and salsa.

12. Chickpea and Spinach Coconut Curry:
   - Simmer chickpeas and spinach in a coconut milk-based curry sauce. Serve over rice.

13. Eggplant and Zucchini Lasagna:
   - Create layers of thinly sliced eggplant and zucchini with dairy-free ricotta. Bake until bubbly.

14. Teriyaki Chicken Skewers with Pineapple Quinoa:
   - Skewer teriyaki-marinated chicken with pineapple chunks. Serve over pineapple-infused quinoa.

15. Stuffed Acorn Squash with Quinoa and Cranberries:
   - Roast acorn squash halves stuffed with quinoa, cranberries, and pecans.

16. Mushroom and Spinach Risotto:
   - Make a creamy dairy-free risotto using mushrooms, spinach, and vegetable broth.

17. Baked BBQ Chicken with Sweet Potato Fries:
   - Coat chicken in gluten-free BBQ sauce and bake. Serve with homemade sweet potato fries.

18. Coconut Lime Shrimp Tacos with Jicama Tortillas:
   - Sauté shrimp in coconut lime sauce. Serve in jicama slices as taco shells.

19. Moroccan Lamb Tagine with Cauliflower Couscous:
   - Slow-cook lamb with Moroccan spices. Serve over cauliflower couscous.

20. Sweet and Sour Tofu with Quinoa:
   - Coat tofu in a sweet and sour sauce. Serve over a bed of cooked quinoa.

More tips for Gluten-Free and Dairy-Free Cooking:
Gluten-Free Flour Alternatives:
   - Utilize almond flour, coconut flour, or rice flour in place of wheat flour for various recipes.

Dairy-Free Substitutes:
   - Substitute coconut milk, almond milk, or cashew cream for dairy milk or cream.

Gluten-Free Condiments:
   - Choose gluten-free soy sauce, tamari, and Worcestershire sauce.

Fresh Herbs and Spices:
   - Enhance flavors with fresh herbs, spices, and citrus to compensate for the absence of dairy.

Nutritional Yeast:
   - To give food a cheesy flavor, add nutritional yeast.

Read Labels:
   - Be vigilant about hidden gluten or dairy in processed foods. Opt for products labeled gluten-free and dairy-free.

By exploring these recipes, you can enjoy a diverse range of gluten-free and dairy-free dinners while savoring a variety of flavors and textures.

CHAPTER SIX

Deserts

Creating delicious gluten-free and dairy-free desserts is a delightful endeavor that allows for indulgence without compromising on dietary preferences. Here's a comprehensive guide along with some mouth-watering recipes:

Base Ingredients:
1. Gluten-Free Flours:
    - Almond flour, coconut flour, rice flour, and gluten-free oat flour are popular choices.

2. Natural Sweeteners:
    - Opt for maple syrup, honey, agave nectar, or coconut sugar as alternatives.

3. Dairy-Free Fats:
    - Coconut oil, avocado oil, and nut butters replace traditional butter in many recipes.

4. Egg Replacements:
    - Use flax eggs (ground flaxseed mixed with water), applesauce, or mashed bananas.

Recipe Ideas:
1. Almond Flour Chocolate Chip Cookies:

- Combine almond flour, coconut oil, and dairy-free chocolate chips for chewy, gluten-free cookies.

2. Coconut Flour Lemon Bars:
   - Create a gluten-free crust using coconut flour and top it with a zesty lemon filling.

3. Chocolate Avocado Mousse:
   - Blend ripe avocados, cocoa powder, and sweetener for a rich and creamy mousse.

4. Gluten-Free Banana Bread:
   - Use gluten-free flour and mashed bananas for a moist and flavorful banana bread.

5. Raspberry Almond Tart:
   - Make an almond flour crust and fill it with dairy-free almond cream and fresh raspberries.

6. Chia Seed Pudding:
   - Mix chia seeds with coconut milk, sweetener, and vanilla for a simple, nutritious pudding.

7. Gluten-Free Apple Crisp:
   - Top sliced apples with a gluten-free crumble made with oats, almond flour, and coconut oil.

8. Cashew Coconut Bliss Balls:
   - Blend cashews, shredded coconut, dates, and a touch of vanilla. Roll into bite-sized bliss balls.

9. Avocado Chocolate Truffles:
   - Blend ripe avocados with cocoa powder and sweetener. Roll into truffles and coat with shredded coconut or chopped nuts.

10. Dairy-Free Ice Cream:
   - Make ice cream using coconut milk or almond milk as the base. Add fruit, chocolate, or vanilla to flavor it.

11. Gluten-Free Lemon Cupcakes:
   - Bake gluten-free lemon cupcakes and top them with dairy-free frosting made with coconut cream.

12. Peanut Butter Chocolate Bars:
   - Layer gluten-free oat and peanut butter base with dairy-free chocolate ganache.

13. Blueberry Almond Cake:
   - Combine almond flour with fresh blueberries for a gluten-free and dairy-free cake.

14. Dairy-Free Rice Pudding:
   - Cook rice in coconut milk, sweeten it, and add a touch of cinnamon for a comforting dessert.

15. Chocolate Coconut Popsicles:
   - Blend coconut milk and cocoa powder, freeze in molds for refreshing dairy-free popsicles.

Tips for Gluten-Free and Dairy-Free Baking:
Texture Enhancers:
   - Add ingredients like xanthan gum or ground flaxseed to enhance the texture of gluten-free baked goods.

Nut and Seed Flours:
   - Experiment with almond, coconut, or hazelnut flours for a variety of flavors in your desserts.

Dairy-Free Whipped Cream:
   - Coconut whipped cream is an excellent dairy-free alternative for topping desserts.

Gluten-Free Baking Powder:
   - Ensure your baking powder is gluten-free, or make your own using cream of tartar and baking soda.

Frozen Fruits:
   - Use frozen fruits in desserts like smoothies, sorbets, or fruity ice creams.

Creating gluten-free and dairy-free desserts opens the door to a world of delightful flavors and textures. Experiment with these base ingredients and recipes to discover the joy of sweet treats that align with your dietary preferences.

CHAPTER SEVEN

Soup, Seafood and Snacks

Soup

Crafting gluten-free and dairy-free soups allows you to savor comforting and flavorful bowls while adhering to dietary preferences. Here's a comprehensive guide along with some delicious recipes:

Base Ingredients:
1. Gluten-Free Broths:
    - Use gluten-free vegetable, chicken, or beef broths as the base for soups.
2. Gluten-Free Grains:
    - Quinoa, rice, gluten-free pasta, or rice noodles are excellent gluten-free options.
3. Vegetables:
   - A variety of fresh or frozen vegetables can add color, flavor, and nutrition.
4. Proteins:
    - Lean meats, poultry, tofu, or legumes can provide protein without gluten or dairy.
5. Dairy-Free Creaminess:
    - Coconut milk, almond milk, or cashew cream can replace traditional dairy for a creamy texture.

Soup Recipes:
1. Gluten-Free Chicken and Rice Soup:
   - Simmer chicken, rice, carrots, celery, and onions in gluten-free chicken broth until tender.

2. Dairy-Free Tomato Basil Soup:
   - Sauté tomatoes, onions, and garlic. Blend with basil and vegetable broth for a luscious dairy-free tomato soup.

3. Quinoa and Vegetable Stew:
   - Combine quinoa, a mix of vegetables, and gluten-free vegetable broth for a hearty stew.

4. Lentil and Spinach Soup:
   - Cook lentils with spinach, carrots, and spices in a gluten-free vegetable broth.

5. Coconut Curry Butternut Squash Soup:
   - Roast butternut squash, blend with coconut milk, and curry spices for a creamy soup.

6. Mexican Chicken Tortilla Soup:
   - Simmer shredded chicken, black beans, corn, and tomatoes in gluten-free chicken broth. Top with gluten-free tortilla strips.

7. Gluten-Free Minestrone Soup:
   - Combine gluten-free pasta, tomatoes, beans, and vegetables in a flavorful vegetable broth.

8. Creamy Broccoli and Potato Soup:
   - Cook potatoes and broccoli in a gluten-free vegetable broth. Blend until creamy and season.

9. Thai Coconut Noodle Soup:
   - Cook rice noodles, vegetables, and tofu in a coconut milk-based broth with Thai spices.

10. Spicy Black Bean Soup:
   - Simmer black beans, tomatoes, corn, and spices in gluten-free vegetable broth for a hearty soup.

11. Gluten-Free Italian Wedding Soup:
   - Make gluten-free meatballs using ground meat and rice crumbs. Add to a broth with vegetables and gluten-free pasta.

12. Dairy-Free Mushroom Soup:
   - Sauté mushrooms, onions, and garlic. Blend with almond milk for a creamy, dairy-free mushroom soup.

13. Moroccan Chickpea Soup:
   - Cook chickpeas, tomatoes, and spices in gluten-free vegetable broth. Finish with fresh herbs.

14. Sweet Potato and Coconut Soup:
   - Roast sweet potatoes and blend with coconut milk, ginger, and spices for a creamy soup.

15. Gluten-Free Clam Chowder:
   - Use gluten-free flour and coconut milk to create a creamy clam chowder.

Tips for Gluten-Free and Dairy-Free Soups:

Thickeners:
 - Use gluten-free flours like rice flour or cornstarch for thickening soups.

Gluten-Free Pasta:
   - Opt for gluten-free pasta or rice noodles for pasta-based soups.

Herbs and Spices:
   - Enhance flavors with herbs and spices to compensate for the absence of dairy.

Dairy-Free Garnishes:
   - Top soups with dairy-free alternatives like coconut yogurt or chopped nuts.

Read Labels:
   - Check labels for hidden gluten in broths and flavorings.

- Homemade Broths:
   - Consider making homemade broths to ensure they are gluten-free.

By incorporating these base ingredients and recipes, you can enjoy a variety of flavorful and nourishing gluten-free and dairy-free soups. Experiment with different combinations to find your favorite comforting bowl.

Seafood

Creating gluten-free and dairy-free seafood dishes opens up a world of delicious and nutritious options. Here's a comprehensive guide along with some mouth-watering recipes:

Base Ingredients:

1. Fresh Seafood:
   - Opt for a variety of fresh fish, shrimp, scallops, clams, and mussels.

2. Gluten-Free Marinades and Sauces:
   - Use gluten-free soy sauce, tamari, or other gluten-free marinades and sauces.

3. Healthy Fats:
   - Incorporate olive oil, coconut oil, or avocado oil for cooking.

4. Herbs and Citrus:
   - Enhance flavors with fresh herbs, garlic, and citrus like lemon or lime.

5. Gluten-Free Grains:
   - Serve seafood over gluten-free grains like quinoa, rice, or gluten-free pasta.

Seafood Recipes:
1. Grilled Lemon Garlic Shrimp:
   - Marinate shrimp in a mixture of garlic, lemon, and olive oil, then grill until cooked.

2. Baked Lemon Herb Cod:
   - Season cod fillets with herbs and lemon, then bake until flaky.

3. Coconut Lime Salmon:
   - Coat salmon with a mix of coconut milk, lime, and spices before baking or grilling.

4. Gluten-Free Fish Tacos:
   - Use corn tortillas and top them with grilled or baked fish, cabbage slaw, and dairy-free sauce.

5. Garlic Butter Shrimp with Zoodles:
   - Sauté shrimp in garlic and dairy-free butter, serve over zucchini noodles.

6. Lemon Dill Baked Scallops:
   - Bake scallops with a lemon-dill marinade until tender.

7. Thai Basil Coconut Mussels:
   - Cook mussels in a Thai-inspired broth with coconut milk, basil, and chili.

8. Gluten-Free Shrimp Scampi:

- Sauté shrimp in olive oil, garlic, and white wine. Serve over gluten-free pasta.

9. Grilled Swordfish Steaks:
   - Marinate swordfish steaks in a mix of herbs and grill until done.

10. Mango Salsa Tuna Steaks:
    - Top seared tuna steaks with a refreshing mango salsa.

11. Sesame Ginger Glazed Salmon:
    - Glaze salmon with a mixture of sesame oil, ginger, and gluten-free soy sauce. Bake or grill.

12. Scallops and Asparagus Stir-Fry:
    - Stir-fry scallops and asparagus in a gluten-free teriyaki sauce.

13. Cajun Grilled Shrimp Skewers:
    - Skewer shrimp with Cajun spices and grill for a flavorful dish.

14. Gluten-Free Seafood Paella:
    - Create a gluten-free paella with a variety of seafood, saffron, and rice.

15. Lemon Pepper Baked Halibut:
    - Season halibut with lemon, pepper, and herbs before baking.

Tips for Gluten-Free and Dairy-Free Seafood Cooking:

Grill or Bake:
   - Choose grilling or baking over frying for a healthier preparation.

Gluten-Free Breading:
  - Use gluten-free breadcrumbs or almond flour for a crispy coating.

Dairy-Free Sauces:
  - Prepare dairy-free sauces using coconut milk, almond milk, or dairy-free butter.

Fresh Citrus:
  - Incorporate fresh citrus like lemon or lime to brighten up seafood flavors.

Gluten-Free Pastas:
   - Opt for gluten-free pasta or grains as accompaniments.

Read Labels:
  - Check labels for hidden gluten in sauces and condiments.

By experimenting with these base ingredients and recipes, you can enjoy a diverse range of flavorful and wholesome gluten-free and dairy-free seafood dishes. Whether grilled, baked, or stir-fried, seafood offers endless possibilities for creating delicious meals that align with your dietary preferences.

Snacks

Creating gluten-free and dairy-free snacks allows for convenient, flavorful, and nutritious options. Here's a comprehensive guide along with some delightful recipes:

Base Ingredients:
1. Gluten-Free Flours:
   - Utilize almond flour, coconut flour, rice flour, or gluten-free oat flour as alternatives.

2. Nut Butters:
   - Almond butter, peanut butter, or cashew butter can add richness and protein.

3. Seeds and Nuts:
   - Incorporate chia seeds, flaxseeds, sunflower seeds, almonds, or walnuts for added texture and nutrients.

4. Fresh Fruits:
   - Include fresh fruits like berries, apples, bananas, or citrus for natural sweetness.

5. Dried Fruits:
   - Add dried fruits such as raisins, apricots, or cranberries for a chewy element.

6. Coconut:
   - Coconut flakes, coconut oil, or coconut milk can contribute a tropical flavor.

Snack Recipes:
1. Energy Bites:
   - Combine dates, nuts, seeds, and gluten-free oats. Shape into small bites for a quick and energizing snack.

2. Homemade Trail Mix:
   - Mix a variety of nuts, seeds, and dried fruits for a customizable and portable snack.

3. Fruit and Nut Bars:
   - Blend dried fruits, nuts, and seeds. Press into a pan and cut into bars for a convenient on-the-go option.

4. Kale Chips:
   - Massage kale leaves with olive oil and seasonings, then bake until crispy for a nutritious alternative to potato chips.

5. Stuffed Dates:
   - Fill dates with nut butter or nuts for a sweet and satisfying snack.

6. Homemade Popcorn:
   - Air-pop popcorn and drizzle with melted coconut oil. For a cheese taste, add nutritional yeast.

7. Vegetable Sticks with Hummus:
   - Slice cucumbers, carrots, and bell peppers. Serve with gluten-free and dairy-free hummus.

8. Chia Pudding Cups:
   - Mix chia seeds with coconut milk and sweetener. Refrigerate until set, then top with fruits.

9. Roasted Chickpeas:
   - Toss chickpeas with olive oil and spices. Roast until crunchy for a protein-packed snack.

10. Frozen Banana Bites:
   - Dip banana slices in dairy-free chocolate and freeze for a sweet frozen treat.

11. Almond Flour Crackers:
   - Combine almond flour, flaxseed meal, and seasonings. Bake into crisp crackers.

12. Sweet Potato Chips:
   - Slice sweet potatoes thinly, toss with coconut oil, and bake for a nutritious alternative to potato chips.

13. Coconut Yogurt Parfait:
   - Layer dairy-free coconut yogurt with granola and fresh berries for a satisfying parfait.

14. No-Bake Granola Bars:
   - Mix gluten-free oats, nuts, seeds, and dried fruits. Press into a pan and refrigerate for easy homemade granola bars.

15. Spiced Roasted Nuts:
   - Toss mixed nuts with spices like cinnamon and paprika. Roast for a flavorful and crunchy snack.

Tips for Gluten-Free and Dairy-Free Snacking:
Read Labels:
   - Check labels for hidden gluten or dairy in packaged snacks.
Portion Control:
   - Be aware of portion quantities to maintain a balanced diet.
Preparation in Batches:
   - Prepare snacks in batches and store them for quick and convenient access.
Hydration:
   - Stay hydrated with water or herbal teas alongside your snacks.
Fresh and Whole Foods:
   - Emphasize fresh, whole foods to ensure a nutrient-rich snacking experience.
Experiment with Flavors:
   - Explore different flavor profiles and spices to keep snacks exciting and satisfying.
By incorporating these base ingredients and recipes, your gluten-free and dairy-free snacks can be both delicious and nourishing, providing a variety of options for different tastes and preferences.

CHAPTER EIGHT

Transitioning to Gluten-Free and Dairy-Free Lifestyle

Transitioning to a gluten-free and dairy-free lifestyle can be both empowering and rewarding for your health. Here's a comprehensive guide to help you make a smooth and successful transition:

Understanding the Basics:
1. Educate Yourself:
   - Learn about gluten and dairy sources. Gluten is found in wheat, barley, and rye, while dairy includes milk, cheese, and yogurt.

2. Label Reading:
   - Get in the habit of reading food labels. Look for gluten and dairy derivatives, and be aware of hidden ingredients.

Assessing Your Current Diet:
3. Food Diary:
   - Keep a food diary to understand your current dietary habits. Identify gluten and dairy-containing items you commonly consume.

4. Identify Alternatives:
   - Research and compile a list of gluten-free and dairy-free alternatives. Familiarize yourself with alternative flours, grains, and dairy substitutes.

Kitchen Transition:
5. Kitchen Cleanout:
   - Conduct a kitchen cleanout. Remove items containing gluten and dairy to create a clean slate.

6. Stocking Essentials:
   - Stock up on gluten-free flours, alternative grains (quinoa, rice), gluten-free pasta, and dairy alternatives (almond milk, coconut milk).

Meal Planning and Prepping:
7. Plan Balanced Meals:
   - Plan balanced meals with a variety of fruits, vegetables, lean proteins, and gluten-free grains. This ensures nutritional adequacy.

8. Batch Cooking:
   - Embrace batch cooking to simplify meal preparation. For convenience, cook in bulk and freeze portions.

Navigating Social Situations:
9. Communication:
   - Communicate your dietary needs to friends, family, and restaurants. Clear communication helps in avoiding unintentional gluten or dairy exposure.

10. Restaurant Strategies:
   - Research restaurants with gluten-free and dairy-free options. Call ahead to inquire about their menu and food preparation practices.

Managing Cravings and Emotional Aspects:
11. Explore Alternatives:
   - Discover gluten-free and dairy-free alternatives for your favorite dishes. There are often delicious substitutes available.

12. Mindful Eating:
   - Practice mindful eating to savor and appreciate the flavors of your new choices. This can help manage cravings.

Seeking Professional Guidance:
13. Consult with a Nutritionist:
   - Consider consulting with a nutritionist or dietitian, especially if you have specific health conditions or concerns. They can provide personalized guidance.

14. Healthcare Provider Consultation:
   - If you suspect gluten sensitivity or celiac disease, consult with a healthcare provider for proper testing and diagnosis.

Staying Positive and Motivated:
15. Celebrate Successes:

- Celebrate your successes, no matter how small. Each step is a positive move towards a healthier lifestyle.

16. Connect with a Community:
   - Join online communities or local support groups for individuals following a gluten-free and dairy-free lifestyle. Experiences and advice from others can be very helpful.

Monitoring Health and Adjusting:
17. Listen to Your Body:
   - Pay attention to how your body responds to the changes. Monitor energy levels, digestion, and overall well-being.

18. Adjustments Over Time:
   - Understand that adjustments may be needed over time. Your preferences and dietary needs may evolve.

Final Thoughts:
Transitioning to a gluten-free and dairy-free lifestyle is a gradual process. Be patient with yourself, and view it as an opportunity to explore new flavors and culinary experiences. With careful planning, a positive mindset, and support from professionals and communities, you can successfully embrace this lifestyle for improved health and well-being.

CHAPTER NINE

Balanced Diets

Eating a balanced diet is essential for good health and wellbeing in general. Eating a balanced diet guarantees that your body gets the proper amounts of vital nutrients. When following a gluten-free and dairy-free lifestyle, it becomes even more important to pay attention to obtaining key nutrients from alternative sources. Here's a comprehensive guide on the importance of a balanced diet and sources of key nutrients in gluten-free and dairy-free options:

Importance of a Balanced Diet:
1. Nutrient Variety:
   - A balanced diet provides a wide array of nutrients, including carbohydrates, proteins, fats, vitamins, and minerals, which are essential for various bodily functions.

2. Energy Maintenance:
   - Balancing macronutrients helps maintain energy levels, supporting daily activities and overall vitality.

3. Weight Management:
   - A balanced diet contributes to weight management by ensuring that you consume the right amount of calories without excessive intake of unhealthy fats or sugars.

4. Optimal Health:

- Nutrient-rich foods promote optimal health, strengthen the immune system, and reduce the risk of chronic diseases.

5. Digestive Health:

- A variety of fibers from different food sources supports digestive health, preventing issues like constipation and promoting a healthy gut microbiome.

Sources of Key Nutrients in Gluten-Free Options:

1. Protein:

- Sources: Lean meats, poultry, fish, eggs, legumes, tofu, and quinoa.
- Gluten-Free Alternatives: Quinoa, lentils, chickpeas, beans, and gluten-free plant-based protein sources.

2. Fiber:

- Sources: Whole grains, fruits, vegetables, and legumes.
- Gluten-Free Alternatives: Brown rice, quinoa, gluten-free oats, sweet potatoes, and a variety of fruits and vegetables.

3. Calcium:

-Sources: Dairy products, leafy greens, almonds, and fortified foods.

-Dairy-Free Alternatives: Fortified plant-based milks (almond, soy, coconut), leafy greens (kale, collard greens), and fortified cereals.

4. Vitamin D:
   -Sources: Sunlight, fatty fish, egg yolks, and fortified dairy products.
   -Dairy-Free Alternatives: Fortified plant-based milk, orange juice, and supplements if needed.

5. Iron:
   -Sources: Red meat, poultry, fish, beans, lentils, and dark leafy greens.
   - Gluten-Free Alternatives: Quinoa, lentils, beans, fortified gluten-free cereals, and dark leafy greens.

Sources of Key Nutrients in Dairy-Free Options:
1. Calcium:
   -Sources: Dairy alternatives fortified with calcium, leafy greens, almonds, and chia seeds.

2. Vitamin B12:
   -Sources: Fish, meat, poultry, eggs, and dairy products.
   -Dairy-Free Alternatives: Fortified plant-based milk, nutritional yeast, and B12 supplements if needed.

3. Omega-3 Fatty Acids:
   -Sources: walnuts, flaxseeds, chia seeds, and fatty fish (mackerel, salmon).

-Dairy-Free Alternatives: Plant-based omega-3 supplements, chia seeds, flaxseeds, and algae-based supplements.

4. Probiotics:
   -Sources: Yogurt, kefir, and fermented dairy products.
   -Dairy-Free Alternatives: Fermented plant-based products like coconut yogurt or sauerkraut.

Tips for a Balanced Gluten-Free and Dairy-Free Diet:

1. Diversify Your Plate:
   - Include a variety of fruits, vegetables, whole grains, and proteins in each meal.

2. Read Labels:
   - Be vigilant about reading labels to ensure that gluten-free and dairy-free alternatives are fortified with essential nutrients.

3. Consider Supplements:
   - If certain nutrients are challenging to obtain from food sources, consider consulting a healthcare provider for appropriate supplements.

4. Stay Hydrated:
   - Water is necessary for healthy digestion and general wellbeing. Ensure an adequate intake of fluids throughout the day.

5. Consult a Nutritionist:
   - Seek guidance from a nutritionist or dietitian to tailor a balanced gluten-free and dairy-free meal plan based on individual needs.

A balanced diet, rich in nutrients from a variety of sources, forms the foundation for a healthy lifestyle, even when navigating gluten-free and dairy-free options. By incorporating a diverse range of nutrient-dense foods, you can promote overall well-being and thrive on your chosen dietary path.

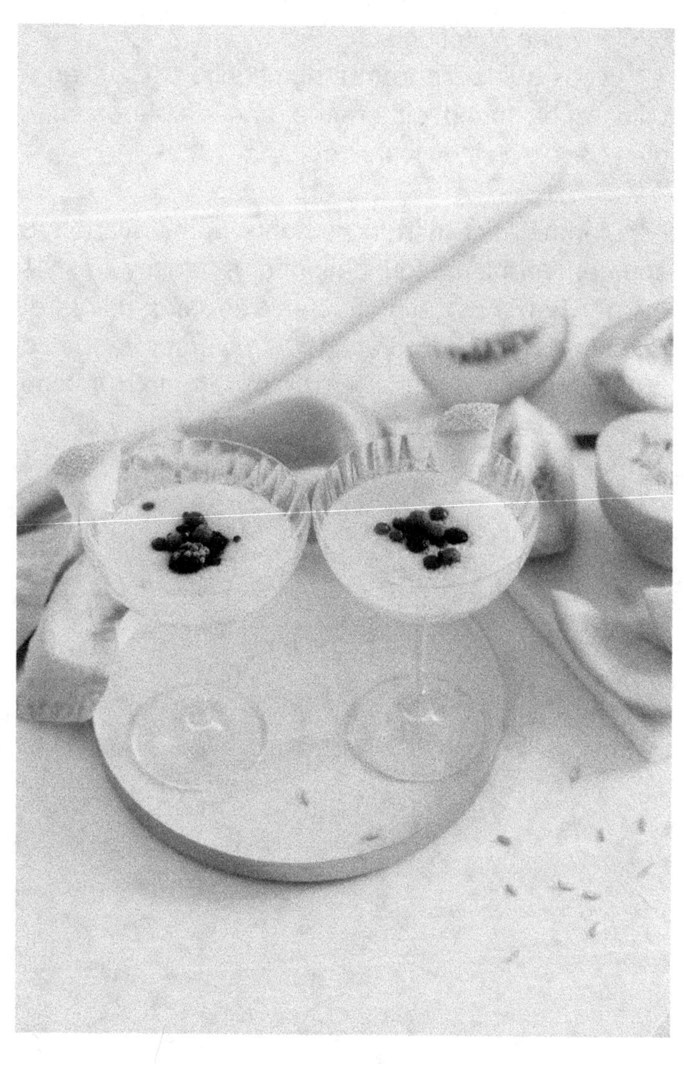

CHAPTER TEN

Health Considerations

Health considerations play a crucial role when adopting dietary changes, particularly in the context of a gluten-free and dairy-free lifestyle. Here's a comprehensive guide on health considerations associated with these dietary choices:

Celiac Disease and Gluten Sensitivity:
1. Celiac Disease:
   -Definition: An autoimmune disorder where the ingestion of gluten leads to damage in the small intestine.
   -Health Considerations: Untreated celiac disease can result in malabsorption of nutrients, leading to deficiencies, digestive issues, and long-term complications.

2. Non-Celiac Gluten Sensitivity:
   - Definition: Individuals experience gluten-related symptoms without the autoimmune response seen in celiac disease.
   - Health Considerations: Symptoms may include digestive issues, fatigue, headaches, and joint pain. It's crucial to manage symptoms through a gluten-free diet.

Lactose Intolerance and Dairy Allergies:
3. Lactose Intolerance:

- Definition: Inability to digest lactose, the sugar found in milk.

- Health Considerations: Symptoms include bloating, gas, and diarrhea. Choosing dairy-free alternatives can help manage these symptoms.

4. Dairy Allergies:

-Definition: An allergic reaction to proteins in cow's milk.

-Health Considerations: Allergic reactions can range from mild to severe. Avoiding dairy is essential, and substitutes like almond or soy milk can be used.

Nutrient Deficiencies:

5. Calcium Deficiency:

- Health Considerations: Dairy is a primary source of calcium. Ensure adequate intake through fortified dairy-free alternatives, leafy greens, and supplements if needed.

6. Vitamin D Deficiency:

-Health Considerations: Limited exposure to sunlight and reduced dairy intake may lead to vitamin D deficiency. Consider fortified plant-based milk and supplements.

7. B12 Deficiency:

-Health Considerations: Common in a vegan diet. Include B12-fortified foods or supplements to prevent anemia and neurological issues.

8. Iron Deficiency:
-Health Considerations: Gluten-free and dairy-free diets may lack iron-rich foods. Include lean meats, lentils, and fortified gluten-free cereals to prevent anemia.

Gastrointestinal Health:
9. Fiber Intake:
-Health Considerations: Gluten-free diets may lack fiber without whole grains. Include gluten-free fiber sources like fruits, vegetables, and gluten-free grains.

10. Probiotics:
-Health Considerations: Reduced intake of fermented dairy may impact gut health. Include dairy-free probiotics or fermented plant-based products.

Digestive Health and Gut Microbiome:
11. Gluten and Gut Health:
Health Considerations: For individuals with gluten sensitivity, avoiding gluten supports gut health by preventing inflammation and maintaining the balance of gut bacteria.

12. Dairy and Gut Health:
- Health Considerations: Some individuals may experience improved digestion by avoiding dairy, especially if lactose intolerant.

Weight Management:
13. Gluten-Free and Dairy-Free Diets for Weight Loss:
    -Health Considerations: While these diets can contribute to weight loss, it's essential to ensure a balanced intake of nutrients and avoid overly processed gluten-free and dairy-free products.

Overall Well-Being:
14. Energy Levels:
    -Health Considerations: Ensure sufficient intake of macronutrients and micronutrients for sustained energy levels. Adjust diet as needed.

15. **Skin Health**:
   -Health Considerations: Some individuals report improved skin health when eliminating gluten and dairy. Monitor skin reactions and consult a dermatologist if needed.

Consulting Healthcare Professionals:
16. Nutritional Guidance:
    -Health Considerations: Consult with a registered dietitian or nutritionist for personalized guidance, especially if managing specific health conditions.

17. Medical Advice:
        -Health Considerations: Before making significant dietary changes, consult with healthcare professionals to ensure these choices align with individual health needs.

In conclusion, health considerations in a gluten-free and dairy-free lifestyle are multifaceted. While these diets can be beneficial for certain conditions, it's essential to approach them mindfully, addressing potential nutrient deficiencies, and seeking guidance from healthcare professionals for optimal health outcomes. Individual responses to these dietary changes vary, and a balanced approach is key to achieving overall well-being.

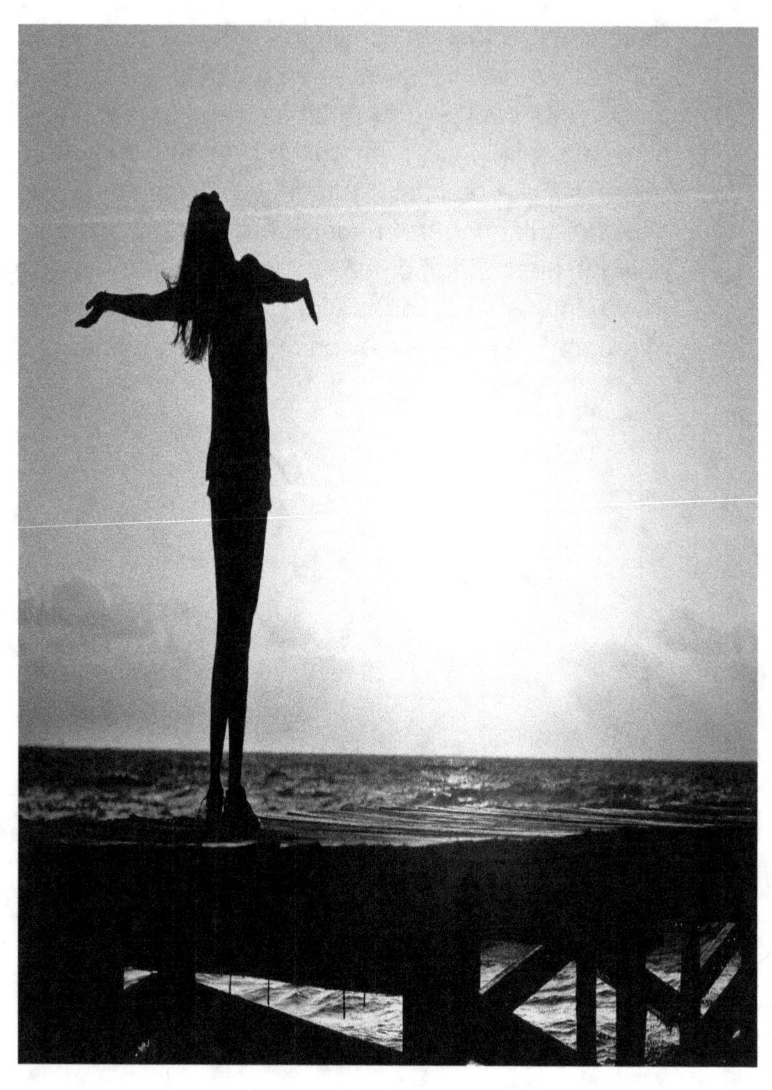

CHAPTER ELEVEN

Allergy Alerts

Allergy alerts are critical components of any dietary lifestyle, particularly for individuals following a gluten-free and dairy-free regimen. Being aware of potential allergens is essential for preventing adverse reactions. Here's a comprehensive guide on allergy alerts in the context of gluten-free and dairy-free living:

1. **Gluten Allergy Alerts**:

1.1 Celiac Disease:
   - Alerts: Individuals with celiac disease must strictly avoid gluten-containing grains like wheat, barley, and rye.
   -Cross-Contamination Risk: Cross-contamination in food preparation can trigger reactions. Gluten-free kitchen practices are vital.

1.2 Gluten Sensitivity:
   - Alerts: People with non-celiac gluten sensitivity need to be vigilant about hidden gluten in processed foods.
   -Label Reading: Constantly reading labels to identify gluten and its derivatives is crucial.

2. **Dairy Allergy Alerts**:

2.1 Lactose Intolerance:

- Alerts: Individuals with lactose intolerance must avoid foods containing lactose, the sugar in milk.

-Dairy-Free Alternatives: Awareness of dairy-free alternatives and reading labels for hidden lactose is essential.

2.2 Dairy Allergies:

- Alerts: Those with dairy allergies need to avoid all forms of cow's milk, including hidden ingredients in processed foods.

-Cross-Contamination Risk: Cross-contamination in kitchens or at restaurants is a concern.

3. **Hidden Ingredients**:
3.1 Gluten:

- Alerts: Gluten can hide in unexpected places such as sauces, dressings, and even medications.

-Education: Constant education on hidden sources is necessary for those with gluten-related issues.

3.2 Dairy:

- Alerts: Dairy derivatives like whey and casein can be present in processed foods.

-Reading Labels: Scrutinizing labels for dairy-related ingredients is crucial.

4. **Cross-Contamination Awareness:**
4.1 Gluten Cross-Contamination:

- Alerts: Cross-contamination can occur in shared kitchens, toasters, or cooking utensils.

-Safe Cooking Practices: Awareness of safe cooking practices to prevent cross-contamination is vital.

4.2 Dairy Cross-Contamination:
  - Alerts: Shared surfaces and equipment can lead to dairy cross-contamination.
  -Communication: Clear communication with restaurants and food establishments is crucial to avoid cross-contact.

5. **Hidden Gluten in Medications**:
5.1 Medication Ingredients:
  - **Alerts:** Some medications may contain gluten as a filler or binding agent.
  -Pharmacist Consultation: Consulting with a pharmacist to ensure medications are gluten-free is important.

6. **Allergen Labeling:**
6.1 Gluten-Free Labeling:
  -Alerts: Products labeled gluten-free can still pose a risk due to cross-contamination.
  -Certification: Some individuals prefer products with gluten-free certifications for added assurance.

6.2 Dairy-Free Labeling:
  - **Alerts:** Products labeled dairy-free may still contain traces of dairy.
  - **Reading Labels:** Reading labels carefully and verifying dairy-free status is essential.

7. **Restaurant Awareness:**
7.1 Menu Inquiry:

- **Alerts:** Many restaurant dishes may contain hidden gluten or dairy.

- Communication: Inquiring about ingredients and informing servers about dietary restrictions is crucial.

8. **Emergency Preparedness:**
8.1 Allergy Emergency Kit:

- Alerts: Carrying an allergy emergency kit with necessary medications is vital for unforeseen circumstances.

- Communication: Informing close contacts about allergies and emergency procedures is important.

9. **Support Networks**:
9.1 Community Engagement:

- Alerts: Joining gluten-free and dairy-free communities can provide valuable insights and support.

- Shared Experiences: Sharing experiences with others navigating similar dietary challenges can be empowering.

10. **Regular Health Checkups**:
10.1 Monitoring Health:

-Alerts: Regular health checkups help monitor overall health and address any arising issues promptly.

- Health Professional Consultation: Consulting healthcare professionals for regular assessments is advisable.

Being vigilant about allergy alerts is a cornerstone of a safe and successful gluten-free and dairy-free lifestyle. This includes continuous education, clear communication, and proactive measures to prevent accidental exposure to allergens. Staying informed, advocating for oneself, and building a supportive network contribute to a positive and healthy experience.

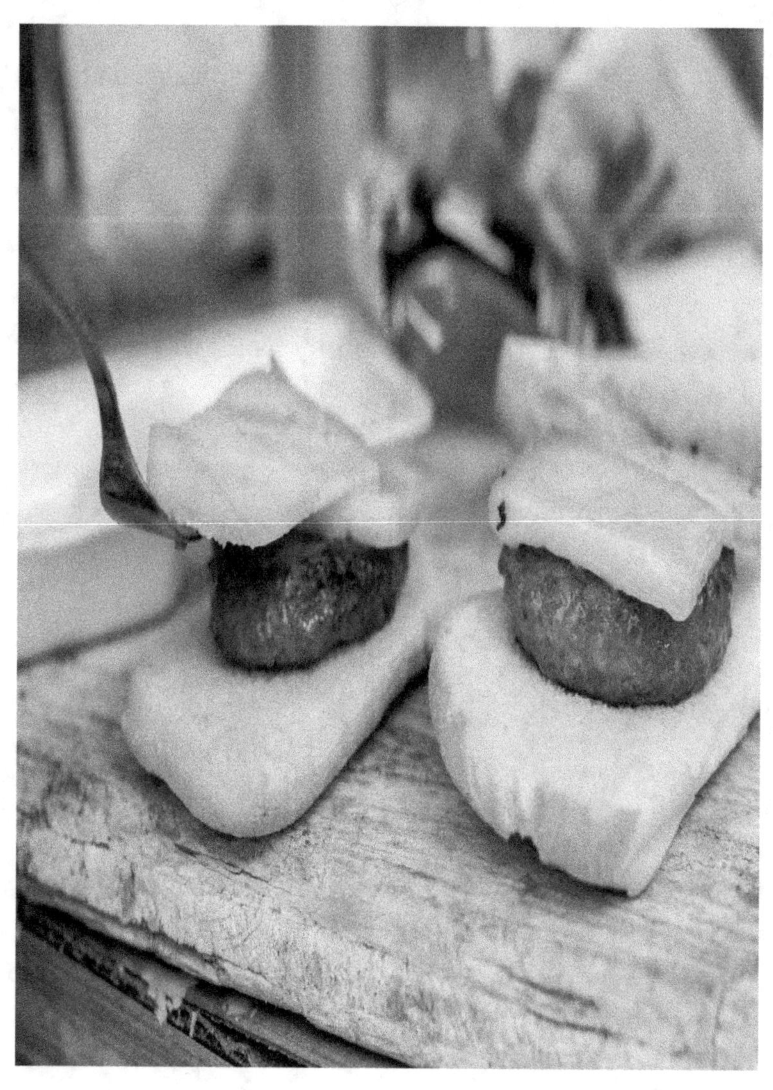

CHAPTER TWELVE

Kitchen Essentials

Equipping your kitchen with the right tools and essentials is essential for successful and enjoyable gluten-free and dairy-free cooking. Here's a comprehensive guide on kitchen essentials for individuals following this dietary lifestyle:

1.Gluten-Free and Dairy-Free Pantry Staples:

1.1 Alternative Flours:
   -Essentials: Almond flour, coconut flour, rice flour, gluten-free oat flour, and quinoa flour.
   - Purpose: Used as substitutes for wheat flour in baking and cooking.

1.2 Gluten-Free Grains:
   - Essentials: Quinoa, rice, millet, buckwheat, and gluten-free oats.
   - Purpose: Serve as versatile alternatives to gluten-containing grains.

1.3 Dairy Alternatives:
   - Essentials: Almond milk, coconut milk, soy milk, and oat milk.
   - Purpose: Substitute for cow's milk in various recipes.

1.4 Gluten-Free Pasta and Noodles:

-Essentials: Rice noodles, corn pasta, quinoa pasta, and other gluten-free options.
 - Purpose: Used in pasta dishes as alternatives to wheat-based options.

1.5 Legumes and Beans:
 - Essentials: Lentils, chickpeas, black beans, and other gluten-free legumes.
 - Purpose: Provide plant-based protein and fiber.

1.6 Gluten-Free Condiments:
 - Essentials: Tamari (gluten-free soy sauce), gluten-free mustard, and gluten-free ketchup.
 -Purpose: Enhance flavor without gluten-containing additives.

1.7 Alternative Sweeteners:
 -Essentials: Maple syrup, honey, agave nectar, and coconut sugar.
 - Purpose: Sweeten dishes without using refined sugars.

2. **Kitchen Equipment**:
2.1 Mixing Bowls:
 - Essentials: Various sizes for mixing batters and ingredients.
 - Purpose: Essential for baking and meal preparation.

2.2 Baking Sheets and Pans:
 - Essentials: Non-stick baking sheets, cake pans, and muffin tins.

- Purpose: Essential for gluten-free baking.

2.3 Blender or Food Processor:
- Essentials: High-quality blender or food processor.
- Purpose: Useful for making smoothies, soups, sauces, and gluten-free flours.

2.4 Stand Mixer or Hand Mixer:
-Essentials: Stand mixer with paddle and whisk attachments or a hand mixer.
- Purpose: Facilitates gluten-free baking and whipping ingredients.

2.5 Food Scale:
- Essentials: Digital food scale.
-Purpose: Ensures accurate measurements for gluten-free and dairy-free baking.

2.6 Knife Set:
- Essentials: Quality chef's knife, paring knife, and serrated knife.
-Purpose: Facilitates precise cutting and chopping of ingredients.

2.7 Cutting Boards:
-Essentials: Separate cutting boards for gluten-free and dairy-free preparation.
-Purpose: Prevents cross-contamination.

2.8 Mixing and Measuring Tools:
  Essentials: Measuring cups, spoons, and silicone spatulas.
  Purpose: Precise measurement and easy mixing.

2.9 Colander:
  -Essentials: Stainless steel or silicone colander.
  -Purpose: Draining gluten-free grains and pasta.

3. Gluten-Free and Dairy-Free Cooking Essentials:

3.1 Herbs and Spices:
  -Essentials: A variety of gluten-free and dairy-free herbs and spices.
  -Purpose: Enhance flavor without relying on gluten-containing seasonings.

3.2 Gluten-Free Baking Powder and Baking Soda:
  -Essentials: Gluten-free baking powder and baking soda.
  -Purpose: Essential leavening agents for gluten-free baking.

3.3 Xanthan Gum or Guar Gum:
  -Essentials: Binders used in gluten-free baking.
  - Purpose: Mimics the elasticity of gluten in baked goods.

3.4 Nutritional Yeast:
  -Essentials: Adds a cheesy flavor to dairy-free dishes.

-Purpose: Commonly used in plant-based recipes.

3.5 Gluten-Free Sauces and Broths:
Essentials: Gluten-free soy sauce, tamari, and gluten-free broths.
 Purpose: Enhance the flavor of dishes.

4. **Storage and Organization:**
4.1 Airtight Containers:
   -Essentials: Glass or BPA-free plastic containers.
   -Purpose: Store gluten-free and dairy-free ingredients safely.

4.2 Labeling System:
   - Essentials: Labels for identifying gluten-free and dairy-free items.
   -Purpose: Prevents accidental consumption of allergens.

4.3 Separate Storage Areas:
   -Essentials: Designate shelves or sections for gluten-free and dairy-free items.
-Purpose: Minimizes the risk of cross-contamination.

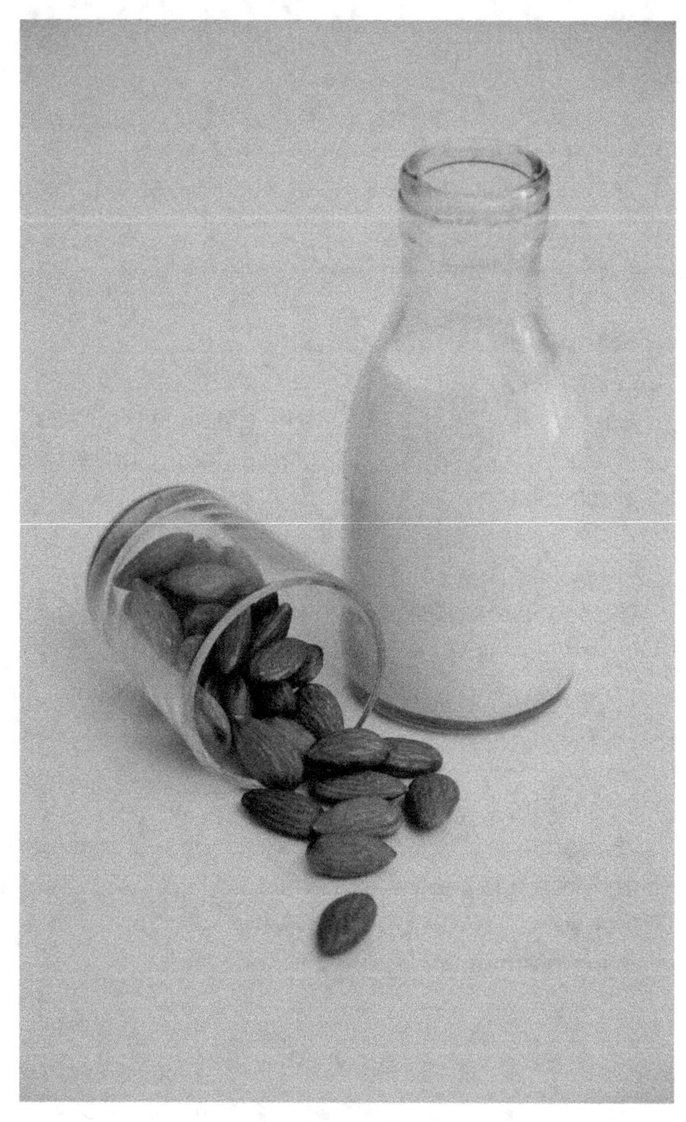

Conclusion

In conclusion, embracing a gluten-free and dairy-free lifestyle is a significant dietary choice that holds various implications for health and well-being. The decision to eliminate gluten and dairy often stems from medical necessity, addressing conditions like celiac disease, gluten sensitivity, lactose intolerance, or dairy allergies. Additionally, some individuals opt for these dietary changes based on personal preferences or a belief in the potential health benefits.

The gluten-free aspect involves avoiding foods containing wheat, barley, and rye, while the dairy-free component necessitates steering clear of products derived from cow's milk. This lifestyle shift requires careful consideration of alternative ingredients, label reading diligence, and informed food choices to ensure nutritional adequacy.

The benefits of adopting a gluten-free and dairy-free lifestyle extend beyond managing specific health conditions. Many individuals report improved energy levels, enhanced digestion, better skin health, and overall well-being. However, it is crucial to approach these dietary changes with mindfulness, ensuring a well-balanced nutritional intake and seeking guidance from healthcare professionals or nutritionists when necessary.

Navigating the gluten-free and dairy-free landscape involves being aware of potential challenges, such as limited food options, cross-contamination risks, and social situations. Overcoming these challenges requires education, strategic planning, and effective communication in various contexts, from grocery shopping to dining out.

Building a gluten-free and dairy-free kitchen involves stocking essential ingredients, utilizing the right kitchen equipment, and implementing thoughtful storage practices to prevent cross-contamination. Educational resources, such as cookbooks and online forums, contribute to culinary creativity and provide valuable insights for individuals embarking on this dietary journey.

Health considerations are paramount in this lifestyle, with a focus on managing conditions like celiac disease, lactose intolerance, and potential nutrient deficiencies. Regular health checkups, dietary adjustments, and staying attuned to individual responses to the dietary changes are essential components of a holistic approach to health.

In the midst of these considerations, it's important to acknowledge the dynamic nature of health and nutrition. What works for one person may not necessarily be suitable for another, emphasizing the need for personalized approaches and ongoing self-assessment.

As individuals navigate the gluten-free and dairy-free terrain, maintaining a positive mindset, celebrating successes, and seeking support from communities and professionals can contribute to a fulfilling and sustainable lifestyle. Ultimately, the gluten-free and dairy-free journey is a continuous exploration, emphasizing the significance of balance, education, and individual well-being in the pursuit of a healthier and happier life.

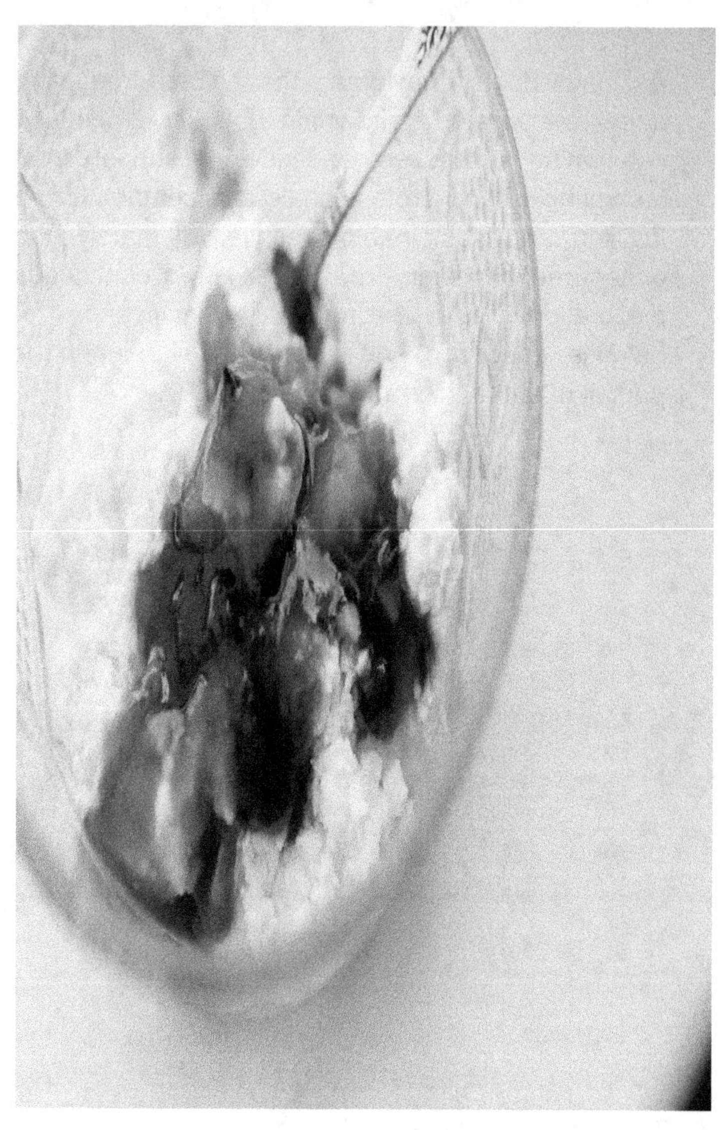